DATE DUE

DEC 12 2008		
	DISCARDED	

Demco, Inc. 38-293

Clinics in Developmental Medicine No. 156
COMMUNICATING WITHOUT SPEECH:
PRACTICAL AUGMENTATIVE AND
ALTERNATIVE COMMUNICATION

© 2001 Mac Keith Press
High Holborn House, 52–54 High Holborn, London WC1V 6RL

Senior Editor: Martin C.O. Bax
Editor: Hilary M. Hart
Managing Editor: Michael Pountney
Sub Editor: Pat Chappelle

First published in this edition 2001

British Library Cataloguing-in-Publication data:
A catalogue record for this book is available from the British Library

ISSN: 0069 4835
ISBN: 1 898683 25 5

Printed by The Lavenham Press Ltd, Water Street, Lavenham, Suffolk
Mac Keith Press is supported by Scope

Clinics in Developmental Medicine No. 156

Communicating Without Speech: Practical Augmentative & Alternative Communication

Edited by

HELEN COCKERILL
Guy's Hospital
London, England

LESLEY CARROLL-FEW
Chelsea & Westminster Hospital
London, England

2001
Mac Keith Press

Distributed 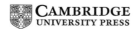 **CAMBRIDGE** UNIVERSITY PRESS

CONTENTS

AUTHORS' APPOINTMENTS   vii

PREFACE   ix

1. THE NEUROLOGY OF SPEECH AND LANGUAGE DISORDERS
   IN CHILDREN. PART I: DISORDERS OF COMPREHENSION
   AND INNER LANGUAGE   1
   J. Keith Brown and Mary E. O'Regan

2. THE NEUROLOGY OF SPEECH AND LANGUAGE DISORDERS IN
   CHILDREN. PART II: DISORDERS OF SPEECH   33
   Mary E. O'Regan and J. Keith Brown

3. WHO NEEDS AUGMENTATIVE COMMUNICATION, AND WHEN?   65
   Martin Bax, Lesley Carroll-Few and Helen Cockerill

4. ASSESSING CHILDREN FOR AUGMENTATIVE AND ALTERNATIVE
   COMMUNICATION   73
   Helen Cockerill and Prue Fuller

5. WORKING WITH FAMILIES TO INTRODUCE AUGMENTATIVE AND
   ALTERNATIVE COMMUNICATION SYSTEMS   88
   *Mats Granlund, Eva Björk-Åkesson, Cecilia Olsson and Bitte
   Rydeman*

6. SUPPORTING CHILDREN USING AUGMENTATIVE AND
   ALTERNATIVE COMMUNICATION IN SCHOOL   103
   Sally Millar

7. THE IMPACT OF ADOLESCENCE ON THE USE OF VOICE OUTPUT
   COMMUNICATION AIDS   124
   Pam Stevenson

8. SUPPORTING AUGMENTATIVE AND ALTERNATIVE
   COMMUNICATION   137
   Susan Balandin and Tessa Barnes-Hughes

9. EXPERIENCES OF CHILDREN AND FAMILIES WHO USE
AUGMENTATIVE AND ALTERNATIVE COMMUNICATION   153
*Compiled by Gillian Hazell, Lesley Carroll-Few and Helen
Cockerill*

10. COMMUNICATION RESOURCES   162
Gillian Hazell and Helen Cockerill

INDEX   179

AUTHORS' APPOINTMENTS

Susan Balandin

Senior Lecturer, School of Communication Sciences and Disorder, The University of Sydney, Sydney, NSW, Australia

Tessa Barnes-Hughes

Manager, Assistive Technology Services, The Spastic Centre of New South Wales, Sydney, NSW, Australia

Martin Bax, DM

Emeritus Reader in Paediatrics, Imperial College of Medicine, Department of Child Health, Chelsea and Westminster Hospital, London, England

Eva Björck-Åkesson

Professor of Education, Mälardalen University, Västerås, Sweden

J. Keith Brown, FRCP

Consultant in Administrative Charge, Departmentt of Paediatric Neurosciences, Royal Hospital for Sick Children; *and* Senior Lecturer, University of Edinburgh, Edinburgh, Scotland

Lesley Carroll-Few, Reg.MRCSLT

Specialist Speech and Language Therapist, Department of Academic Child Health, Chelsea and Westminster Hospital, London, England

Helen Cockerill, BSc, Reg.MRCSLT

Specialist Speech and Language Therapist, Newcomen Centre, Guy's Hospital, London, England

Prue Fuller	*Formerly* Director, ACE Centre; *and* Past President, ISAAC–UK, Oxford, England
Mats Granlund, PhD	Associate Professor of Psychology, Mälardalen University, Västerås; and Research Psychologist, ALA Research Foundation, Stockholm, Sweden
Gillian Hazell, MSc, Reg.MRCSLT	Specialist Speech and Language Therapist, ACE Centre, Oxford, England
Sally Millar, BA, MEd, Reg.MRCSLT	Specialist Speech and Language Therapist and Research Fellow, Communication Aids for Language and Learning (CALL) Centre, University of Edinburgh, Scotland
Cecilia Olsson	Special Educator and Doctoral Student, ALA Research Foundation, Stockholm, Sweden
Mary E. O'Regan, MRCP	Consultant Paediatric Neurologist, Department of Paediatric Neurology, Yorkhill Hospital for Sick Children, Glasgow, Scotland
Bitte Rydeman	Speech Pathologist and Doctoral Student, Göteborg University, Göteborg, and Mälardalen University, Västerås, Sweden
Pam Stevenson, MSc, RegMRCSLT	Head Speech and Language Therapist, Treloar School, Froyle, Hampshire, England

PREFACE

Some children with physical or learning disabilities fail to develop sufficient speech for successful communication. This book identifies other ways in which such children may be enabled to communicate. It describes alternative and augmentative communication (AAC) and is written for doctors and other health professionals who may have no prior knowledge of this field.

Any child at risk of compromised speech development may require AAC systems. These include manual signing, symbol charts and electronic voice-output communication aids.

By presenting current research and accepted good practice in the international field of AAC, authors give detailed information on the neurology of speech and language and provide guidelines for the assessment of non-speaking children. Issues of prognosis for speech, the timing of intervention and the importance of working within a multidisciplinary framework are discussed. The central role of families and schools in the successful introduction of AAC systems and the support necessary for social communication and curriculum access is recognized. The area of literacy and its relationship to AAC systems has not been addressed in detail as the field is felt to be too extensive and specialized to address adequately in the context of this book. The main features of AAC systems and resources are discussed, but readers are directed to local information providers due to the considerable geographical variations both in systems and equipment. Finally, the roles of AAC users and their families are represented in order to emphasize the functional benefit of AAC to children for whom natural speech may not be possible.

LESLEY CARROLL-FEW
HELEN COCKERILL
September 2001

1

THE NEUROLOGY OF SPEECH AND LANGUAGE DISORDERS IN CHILDREN. PART I: DISORDERS OF COMPREHENSION AND INNER LANGUAGE

J. Keith Brown and Mary E. O'Regan

Communication is a two-way process by which information is passed from one person to another. This implies three criteria are met: first, there is some output from the initiating person; second, there is some means of transmitting and conveying the information; and third, the recipient can receive and interpret the information. The usual system is an oral/aural dependent one; a manual/visual system can be used in writing/reading, sign language and pictographs; an oral/visual system is used in lip reading; while in children with severe perceptual disabilities a tactile/tactile system may be the only means of communication. These alternative communication systems will be the subject of the rest of this book; we shall confine ourselves in these opening two chapters to the neurological mechanisms that subserve the oral/aural system and the disorders that disrupt it. Our three criteria can therefore be simplified into an output system for speech, a sound-based language to convey the information, and an aural receptive system that possesses the means of interpreting the language, *i.e.* inner language. Speech is by definition a motor act requiring motor learning. Language has two meanings, which often causes confusion: (1) the symbol system of words and syntax with their phonological equivalents (sound system) and graphic structure (written system); and (2) the semantic or cognitive aspect of *inner language* allowing understanding of the information being transmitted. We will further simplify our task by discussing only the mechanisms of speech production and the neural substrate for understanding, *i.e.* inner language. The characteristics of languages themselves or the rules of social interaction between people, *i.e.* the pragmatics of language use, will not be addressed.

Inner language and cognition
We shall consider inner language before speech development and production, since if a child is not spoken to or cannot hear, then no language or speech will develop. Language is fundamental to thought and intelligence and utilizes most parts of the cerebral cortex. A child may be able to name an object or point to a picture by retrieving the word from her/his lexical store (passive vocabulary); but only if the child can hold the word in short term memory,

1

TABLE 1.1
The neurophysiology and neuropsychology of speech and language development

Section*	Language function	Brain structure discussed
1.1	Peripheral hearing	—
1.2	Central hearing	Heschl's gyrus
1.3	The lexicon	Wernicke's area, planum temporale
1.4	Localization of memories	Cerebral cortex
1.5	Cognition—concept formation	Whole brain
1.6	Symbolic function and inner language	Reticular formation, Wernicke's and Broca's areas, arcuate fasciculus
1.7	Nonverbal communication—emotional overtones	Limbic and extrapyramidal system
2.1	Syntactics	Broca's area, insula
2.2	Phonology	Supplementary area
2.3	Speech production	Pons, medulla

*Items above the dotted line are discussed in this chapter, those below the line in Chapter 2.

while accessing memory banks in all parts of the cerebral cortex that relate to that word, can s/he understand its meaning and so reason. Employing active vocabulary to explain the meaning of a word and so show understanding is a much more sophisticated cognitive task than using simple passive vocabulary. Equally, as age creeps on at the other end of life, naming, *i.e.* nominal recall, becomes more difficult, while understanding is preserved. A primary disorder of inner language therefore has a major effect on global cognitive learning (*i.e.* intelligence).

Most children with a primary language disorder will have associated abnormalities of speech, *i.e.* secondary speech disorders (Ingram 1959), but others will have normal phonological development and be echolalic but without comprehension, *i.e.* a fluent aphasia. This is seen in the echolalia of autism and fragile X syndrome but also in the ability to repeat nursery rhymes and prelearned phrases or even memorize whole conversations. The child has no understanding at all of what s/he is talking about, hence the often applied term of 'cocktail party syndrome'. This is seen particularly in hydrocephalus, hypercalcaemia and Williams syndrome. One has only to look at the real meaning of nursery rhymes used as articulation exercises for toddlers—such as 'Ring-a-ring o' roses' celebrating death from bubonic plague, or 'Goosey goosey gander' making fun of religious intolerance—to see we can all speak without necessarily understanding the meaning of what we say.

A child may therefore have good articulated speech and a severe disorder of inner language, just as s/he may have normal inner language and no speech at all.

While any strict division into input and output or language and speech must be artificial, for present purposes a division is placed between nonverbal communication and syntax, as shown in Table 1.1. The former will be considered in this chapter, and the latter in Chapter 2.

Environmental stimulation
Before considering specific language functions we will describe the environmental conditions

necessary for language learning. If a child is not spoken to s/he will not acquire language, as s/he will not understand nor use words s/he has never heard. The parent is in essence programming a computer, and no matter how good the child's potential, if the quality of speech and language that s/he hears and the sophistication of the grammar and its variety are restricted, this must show in the child's speech and language skills. In addition, frank abuse or neglect has an adverse effect on children's speech and language development (Law and Conway 1992). The number of words in a child's vocabulary rises steeply between 2 and 5 years and is obviously related to the number of different words heard and the sophistication of the grammar. The average adult is thought to have a vocabulary of about 10,000 words. A student may hear up to 100,000 words per day and a highly educated man will have a total vocabulary of 100,000 words. In contrast, it is also suggested that any non-technical idea can be communicated successfully with a basic vocabulary of only 850 words.

The richness of a language environment will be an influential factor in the child's acquisition and use of language skills. Excessive exposure to television, carers who speak the child's home language as a second language, and the frequency of language addressed to the child can all influence the rate and extent of language learning.

It should be remembered that parents will adjust their responses to the child's communication ability, so parents of language-delayed children use simpler sentences and may convey information in a simplified way (Paul and Elwood 1991).

The brain of the human infant at birth is poorly developed as far as cortical function is concerned. The neurons have few dendritic connections, there is practically no myelination of the axons, no association pathways have been formed, and no Nissl substance has been laid down. The brain continues to develop after birth at a very rapid rate, gaining 1000 g in weight during the first four years of life and continuing until around the age of 18 years. The increase in abilities as a result of progressive brain development is the basis of developmental paediatrics. Brain development is dependent not only on genetic factors but also on receiving the appropriate environmental stimulation to ensure the correct dendritic connections. There is mounting evidence that not only is the correct metabolic and nutritional environment necessary but also the brain must receive stimulation of the developing pathways at a particular time in their maturation, *i.e.* during so-called critical or sensitive learning periods.

One optic nerve is more rapidly myelinated if it is stimulated while the other eye is kept covered. According to Blakemore (1974), the actual microscopic anatomy of cerebral cortex subserving vision is determined, once and for all, at the time of rapid postnatal development, dependent upon the type of visual stimulation. If this is true, severe deprivation of environmental stimulation and experience during the first three years of life—i.e. in the critical learning periods—may set up an organic pattern in the brain that cannot later be reversed by increased stimulation. It is thought that a child reared in a linguistically extremely poor environment may not be able to catch up fully, even with intense stimulation, after the age of 6 years (Rutter 1980).

Psychosocial deprivation may arise when the parents are uncaring, unloving, and have little or no bond with their children. A child in such a family is not picked up and cuddled, is fed with a bottle propped up in the pram, and is left with neighbours and siblings. S/he may eventually be abandoned and pass from foster home to foster home or from children's

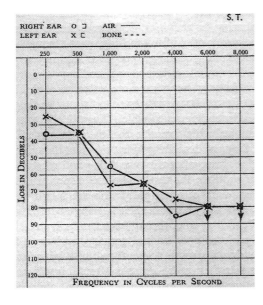

Fig. 1.1. Audiogram in sensorineural deafness showing steep hearing loss between 500 and 2000 Hz that seriously affects perception of consonants in speech.

home to children's home. The clinical picture in severe cases of psychosocial deprivation is of apathy and delayed development in all areas including gross motor function. A positive change in circumstances for young children can result in striking developmental and growth spurts.

Section 1.1—Peripheral hearing

A full assessment of hearing is mandatory in all children with disturbed speech and language development. This must include the minimum decibel thresholds across all the major frequencies (250–8000 Hz). The volume of voice varies within a sentence and also drops dramatically if the person turns away from the listener (*e.g.* the teacher turning to the blackboard), so the normal voice speaking at 60 to 80 dB may be adequate for a child with a mild hearing loss if these fluctuations are minimized by being near and facing the person; however, much meaning is often lost even with a 40 dB loss. Ewing and Taylor, in their Manchester unit, have demonstrated the drastic effect of such losses in children's understanding during play (personal observations). Most children with glue ear have a flat loss around 40 dB, and moderate to severe hearing loss may occur, but severe loss (70–90 dB) and profound loss (>90 dB) are more likely to be sensorineural.

The cochlea responds to specific frequencies along its length and so can be selectively damaged for a particular frequency range. A large organ pipe may have frequencies as low as 20 Hz, while a piccolo or violin may have frequencies audible up to 20,000 Hz. This range of frequency discrimination present for music is not essential for speech. The human ear is most sensitive around 3000 Hz (Fig. 1.1). A hearing loss in the low to middle frequencies (125–2000 Hz) interferes with the perception of vowels and intonation of speech, while the higher frequencies (1500–4000 Hz) affect the consonants. It is the high frequency consonants *s*, *t*, *th* and *sh* that give clarity and easy extraction of meaning of speech. A public address system with a good bass response may make it more difficult to determine where one's train is going than one with a tinny Tannoy. The high frequencies also allow discrimination of the direction of sounds because there are many wavelengths in the distance between the ears, whereas with a low frequency there may be only one. Modern hi-fi equipment utilizes this by having stereo speakers for high frequencies but only a single one for low frequencies.

High frequency hearing loss can be very deceptive as the child may respond to some environmental sounds, but speech will be perceived as rumbly and indistinct. Differentiation of deafness from a dysphasia may then be difficult and takes observation over time to be sure. Amplification in these cases causes already distorted speech to sound even more distorted, so the child will reject hearing aids unless they selectively amplify the high frequencies.

The external ear, the pinna, collects the sound and focuses it onto the tympanic membrane. The relatively large area of the tympanic membrane has its energy focused upon the much smaller oval window; this, plus the mechanical amplification by the lever action of the ossicles—*i.e.* the malleus, incus and stapes—amplifies the sound energy several hundredfold. Middle ear disease may thus have a profound effect on the loudness, but not the frequency, of perceived sound. The stapedius attachment to the round window is controlled by the stapedius muscle, and the stapedius reflex is protective and dampens the sound amplification. This is why if music is loud the whole time one accommodates to it, and a fortissimo is always more effective after a period of pianissimo. Temporary paralysis of this reflex in brainstem disorders such as basilar migraine will cause hyperacusis and phonophobia as sounds appear excessively loud.

CONDUCTIVE DEAFNESS

This is the commonest cause of deafness in children, estimated at 90 per cent of cases, and is usually due to a secretory otitis media (otitis media with effusion—OME). Up to a third of all preschool children will experience at least one episode between 1 and 5 years, the peak age being around 2 years (Zielhuis *et al.* 1989). Over half these episodes will resolve spontaneously within three months, but 10 per cent become chronic, lasting one to four years, and produce a persisting hearing loss of the order of 20–40 dB across all frequencies (Rach *et al.* 1988). The presence of chronic infection causes the mucosa of the middle ear cleft to change, with goblet cell hyperplasia that then results in a persistent sticky secretion. If the adenoids are also enlarged this will prevent drainage of the excess fluid secretion into the middle ear. Diagnosis depends upon a good history, otoscopy with a microscope if necessary for greatest accuracy, impedance audiometry and pure tone audiometry; for absolute proof tympanocentesis is required. The resultant OME, with conductive deafness persisting over months, is now known, as a result of studies in New Zealand and Bristol, to cause slowing of speech development (Abraham *et al.* 1996).

SENSORINEURAL DEAFNESS

The ear develops between the sixth and 14th gestational weeks and is vulnerable to teratogenic congenital infection such as rubella and cytomegalovirus infection. Sensorineural deafness is genetically determined in 50 per cent of cases (Coucke *et al.* 1994); may be of

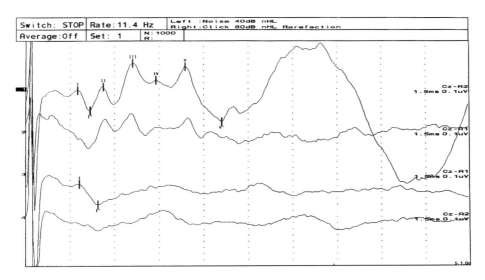

Fig. 1.2. Brainstem evoked response showing peaks for all the brainstem components between cochlea and inferior coliculus in the midbrain.

any mendelian pattern, dominant (one type carried on chromosome 1p), recessive or sex-linked; and can be associated with pigmentary markers such as retinitis pigmentosa, albinism, white nails, white forelock, heterochromia of the iris of the eye, café-au-lait spots or multiple lentigenes. A large number of dysmorphic and metabolic disorders, *e.g.* the Alport, Pendred, Usher and Lange–Nielson syndromes, biotinidase deficiency and the mucopolysacharidoses, are also associated with deafness. Sensorineural deafness may be secondarily acquired due to toxic compounds in the neonatal period, as with bilirubin causing kernicterus, and drugs such as gentamicin, streptomycin and kanamicin. Damage to the VIIIth nerve commonly occurs in the course of bacterial meningitis, *e.g.* 25 per cent of cases with pneumococcus and 9 per cent of those with *Haemophilus influenzae*. Since the cochlea responds to different frequencies in different parts of the spiral structure, damage may be selective, and sensorineural deafness is particularly likely to affect certain frequencies, usually the high ones. Chronic exposure to loud noise is also likely to cause selective cochlea damage affecting the high frequencies. Sensorineural deafness may be congenital or begin after a period of normal hearing, and can be progressive. Hearing impairment due to rubella, for example, may be relatively mild at 1 year but more profound at 4 years as the damage continues postnatally.

Section 1.2—Central hearing

The hard-wiring of the auditory system takes impulses from the cochlea via the VIIIth nerve to the cochlear nucleus. The pathways then decussate and pass via the lateral lemniscus to the inferior colliculus, and then via the medial geniculate nucleus of the thalamus to Heschl's gyrus in the cortex of the temporal lobe. This can be tested using electrocochleography, brainstem evoked responses and cortical auditory evoked responses (Fig. 1.2).

These lower centres are required for auditory reflexes such as startle to a sudden bang, head turn to sound, ducking to a rapidly approaching sound, and localization of sound direction and stereophonic sound.

Localization of sound in space is very accurate within one degree and depends upon a different pathway than speech, involving the superior olives and superior lip of the sylvian fissure. The lateral geniculate nucleus of the thalamus is already specialized for vision in that the large cells of the magnocellular layer receive impulses from the M ganglion cells of the retina and respond to intensity and colour, while the parvocellular system responds to movement and tracking. It is likely that the medial geniculate for hearing is similarly genetically primed for selective acoustic signals such as temporal pattern and frequency. It also has a magnocellular and a parvocellular division; in animals, this has to do with, for instance, birdsong and bats' sonar.

Heschl's gyrus is not visible from the surface of the brain but is very prominent if the superior surface of the temporal lobe is exposed (Fig. 1.3). It theoretically consists of the anterior of the two or three transverse gyri on the superior surface of the temporal lobe. It is thought that there are at least six cochleotopic maps in each Heschl's gyrus area. Each ear is represented in each Heschl's gyrus, and the vestibular part of the VIIIth nerve is adjacent, giving the sensation of rotation. Stimulation of the gyrus causes a roaring, ringing, clicking or buzzing sensation. A bilateral lesion is required to cause deafness, but a unilateral one on the dominant side may cause acquired auditory agnosia. Lesions in the brainstem auditory pathways, e.g. a bilateral lesion in the inferior colliculi, will cause a similar loss of auditory perception to a lesion in Heschl's gyrus (Johkura et al. 1998).

The transverse gyri of Heschl on the left are thought to be responsible for auditory discrimination, e.g. distinguishing sounds with a linguistic meaning from background noise, as well as separating words with minimal phonic differences such as differentiating colour from collar. One also distinguishes acoustic sequences in one's native tongue, even though novel and not previously encountered, so one adds new words to the lexicon and subtracts these from similar tonal sequences in a foreign language and from background noise, tones and music. Those sounds with an emotional connotation, such as intonation indicating boredom, tenderness, anger, sarcasm or happiness, are appreciated on the right. Musical appreciation is also represented in the right Heschl's gyrus, and it is thought that melody, pitch and rhythm are all appreciated separately.

The system is very finely tuned and is able to discriminate between sounds with only a few hertz difference in frequency or milliseconds difference in time, such as ba, ta and da. The time between a consonant and the onset of a voiced vowel is the voice onset time and if less than 20 ms causes a smaller evoked potential in Heschl's gyrus than those of 40 or 60 ms. Proof that these temporal processing parameters are discriminated in Heschl's gyrus, and may pose limitations on speech discrimination, can be demonstrated by looking at auditory evoked potentials when the temporal lobe is exposed during surgery (Steinschneider et al. 1999). In the future, more sophisticated evoked responses, e.g. mismatched negativity and functional MRI and micro-MRI, will further help elucidate function. If speech is too rapid, or differences in duration of a sound too short, this may defeat the system as when first learning a foreign language (rue/roux). Lower frequency sounds as in the vowels and

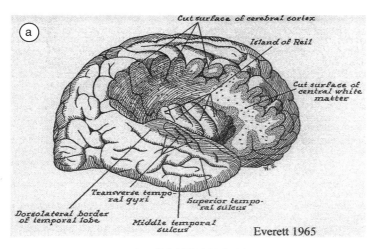

Cut surface of cerebral cortex

Island of Reil

Cut surface of central white matter

Transverse temporal gyri

Superior temporal sulcus

Dorsolateral border of temporal lobe

Middle temporal sulcus

Everett 1965

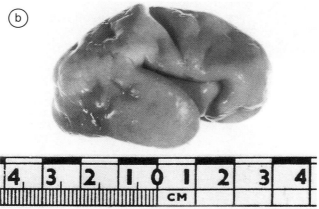

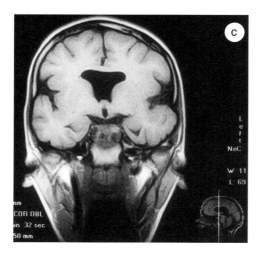

Fig. 1.3. (a) Diagrammatic representation of a cut-away section through the sylvian fissure, showing Heschl's gyrus on the superior surface of the temporal lobe and the large amount of cerebral cortex of the insula normally hidden by the lips (opercula) of the sylvian fissure. (Reproduced by permission from Everett 1965.)

(b) Fetal brain before the lip has closed to show how Broca's area, insular cortex, Heschl's gyrus and Wernicke's area are really contiguous, linked by the external capsule and arcuate fasciculus.

(c) MRI of opercula dysplasia in transverse section with Heschl's gyrus on the superior temporal surface.

8

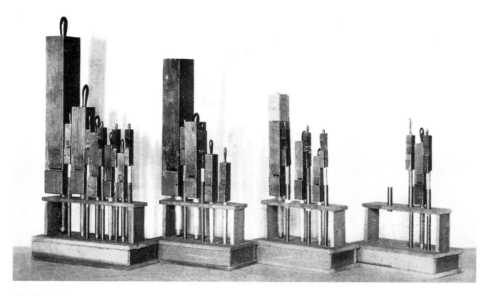

Fig. 1.4. D.C. Miller's organ pipes for the synthetic production of vowel sounds, showing that each vowel requires many pipes and is a composite sound.

short consonants develop in speech before the longer lasting high frequency sounds such as *th* and *sh*, suggesting that the inability to differentiate high frequency or simple duration of sounds is not the main limiting factor in normal speech development but may be very important in abnormal developmental syndromes.

If one attempts to imitate speech sounds by the use of, say, organ pipes, as was tried early last century by D.C. Miller (Ghazala 1993; Fig. 1.4), then one needs several pipes for each sound, *i.e.* they are not simple pure tones. Using speech frequency analysis of phonemes one can see different bands of intensity known as formants. Small variations in the formant structure of individual speech sounds gives us the ability to discriminate similar sounds within words, for example both *s* and *sh* are high-frequency consonants, peaking at up to 7000 Hz, but it is a strong formant band at 2500 Hz in *sh* which separates it from the strong band at 4500 Hz in *s*. It also allows the appreciation of a difference between *oo* and *ee*, due to a formant with *ee* at 2500 Hz. If this is not appreciated, as with high-tone hearing loss, then one cannot differentiate between, for instance, *shoot* and *sheet*.

Sound is bilaterally represented in the brain as neural connections from both ears projected via crossed and uncrossed pathways to the primary auditory cortices in the temporal lobes. The dominant auditory cortex on the left has a predilection for speech as opposed to nonverbal sounds, but if this is damaged in a young child, the opposite side is capable of taking over. All children with a congenital right hemiplegia will usually speak, but 40 per cent will be slow in speech development. Therefore, in congenital word deafness there must be bilateral interference with temporal lobe function. The most common cause is either genetic or due to a bilateral focal cortical dysplasia.

AUDITORY/VERBAL AGNOSIA, CENTRAL DEAFNESS, WORD DEAFNESS,
PHONAGNOSIA

In clinical practice, it may be impossible to distinguish between central word deafness and auditory agnosia (where the association area is affected). As outlined above, both speech and inner language with comprehension will be affected. The pure condition is usually a developmental genetically determined syndrome. Affected children show gross auditory inattention. They hear but cannot listen, and they do not repeat words or phrases nor show echolalia so great care must be taken to exclude a peripheral hearing loss. They do not understand commands but may eventually develop simple passive naming vocabulary. Ability to comprehend language through a visual mode is preserved, and visual ability with drawing, jigsaws, formboards and matching shapes is important to differentiate the disorder from severe learning disability. The children are typically mute or severely dysfluent. If they do speak, their articulation is grossly defective. With pure word deafness the child responds to environmental sounds and may be musical with a good sense of rhythm.

ACQUIRED CENTRAL DEAFNESS AND AUDITORY AGNOSIA

A pure word deafness may follow damage to the superior temporal lobe in older children, and aetiologies include focal tumours, trauma, herpes simplex encephalitis and embolic vascular events. The commonest cause of an auditory agnosia in children is epilepsy in the Landau–Kleffner syndrome, and auditory agnosia is often the initial presenting symptom (Kaga 1999). All children with onset of auditory agnosia (median age around 5 years) should have an EEG, including sleep activation (see below). However, more commonly the lesion is not circumscribed, so the adjacent association area (Wernicke's area) is involved and a receptive dysphasia results. The child loses the ability to understand spoken language (with inability to appreciate the auditory phonemic make-up of words), to repeat sentences, and to write to dictation. When the disorder comes on in the older child, after the acquisition of a lexicon and inner language, there is no deficit in spoken speech or verbal reasoning. The ability to write, read and speak spontaneously is preserved. An adult patient described this beautifully as "Voice comes but no words. I can hear, sounds come, but words don't separate" (Brain 1961). There is a normal response to pure tones and music, but if there is a lesion in the right superior temporal lobe then there is tone deafness with the inability to appreciate musical tones, and this may also involve intonation, *i.e.* a dysprosodia. In pure cases of central word deafness, sign language and lip reading may help, as in the peripherally deaf.

Section 1.3—The lexicon

THE AUDITORY ASSOCIATION AREA

Behind the mountains of Heschl's gyrus is the triangular region of the planum temporale which extends into the superior temporal gyrus (Fig. 1.5). This is the auditory association area and is identical with Wernicke's area. Chimpanzees possess 98 per cent of the same DNA as humans and their brain looks very similar to that of a human, yet they can never speak or develop verbal reasoning. The area of the brain showing the greatest difference between the higher ape and man is the planum temporale. It is preprogrammed to enable

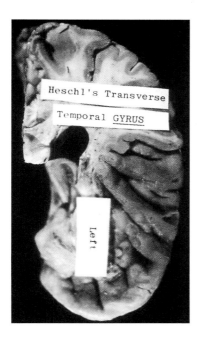

Fig. 1.5. Superior surface of the temporal lobe showing Heschl's transverse gyri anteriorly with the flatter planum temporale behind.

us to learn language; the particular language is not specified, although as Chomski (1972) has suggested, all languages have to possess certain common characteristics (linguistic universals) in order that we can learn them. Sir William Jones (1746–1794) thought that Sanskrit, Latin and Greek had such similarities as to suggest a common source.

The planum temporale, in man, is the most asymmetrical area of the brain and is thought to form the anatomical basis of speech, in particular the lexicon. It is the site of storage of the word dictionary of language. The words are therefore differentiated in Heschl's gyrus and then stored as the brain's dictionary or lexicon in the adjacent planum temporale. If we use a computer analogy, although most software programmes use the computer language, they have to be physically stored somewhere on a hard disk. The computer hardware may also be able to use several languages such as MS Dos, Pascal, Fortran, etc. All human languages, which utilize sound sequences (*i.e.* words), are stored in the planum temporale on the left; tunes and intonation patterns are stored on the right.

The planum temporale is larger and 17 times more cellular on the left (Geschwind and Levitsky 1968). In 100 brains studied by those authors at autopsy, the planum temporale was larger on the left in 65, larger on the right in 11, and of equal size bilaterally in 24. This can now be seen *in vivo* using MRI morphometry. Females show a stronger left-sided planum temporale asymmetry, and function is thought to be determined by early functional differentiation (Preis *et al.* 1999). Heschl's gyrus is longer and often fatter on the left, with a bigger planum temporale. It has been shown that these asymmetries are present *in utero* and are not the effects of language acquisition (Strauss *et al.* 1983). The occipital lobe is wider, the sylvian fissure longer by 6.0mm, and the angular gyrus more prominent on the left side. The axons form thicker myelin sheaths on the left and so white matter volume is greater (Anderson *et al.* 1999).

The pathological basis of such conditions as word deafness, autism and dyslexia is postulated to be a focal dysplasia with ectopic areas of tissue in the planum temporale. Ectopias are areas of abnormal development with neurons in places they should not be such as white matter heterotopias or under the pia mater. The ectopias are mainly sited on the left and along the sylvian fissure and are occasionally overlain by abnormal gyri (Galaburda 1993).

Penfield and Rasmussen (1952) stimulated this area of the brain at neurosurgery in conscious patients. The patients reported hearing music, singing, pianos playing (on stimulation of the right temporal lobe), names being called, street noises, and words and sentences spoken by other voices than their own. This suggested that the superior temporal gyrus and planum contained not only the lexicon, *i.e.* vocabulary, but also engrams of words and sentences as well as the memory bank of sounds heard over years, allowing us for instance to recognize which of our children is speaking. Cerebral blood flow studies using radioactive xenon have demonstrated a definite increase in blood flow to the superior temporal lobe area when listening to words (Nishizawa *et al.* 1982). This area interfaces recognition of words in the planum temporale with conscious awareness in the reticular formation. We 'speak to ourselves' in our heads and hear this in the auditory association area of the temporal lobe. This can now be seen as a focal increase in cerebral blood flow on functional MRI (McGuire *et al.* 1996, Price *et al.* 1994). We do the same whether the source of inner language, that we are currently thinking about in consciousness, arises from peripheral hearing, reading, sign language or abstract reasoning generated within our minds. The ability to realize that words are made up of 46 individual sounds or phonemes (phonological awareness) is also dependent upon this area of brain and is essential for reading and spelling. The localization of sound in space is thought to be separate from the discrimination of words and depends upon the superior lip of the fissure, on the parietal side, related to the body in space.

DIRECT PLANUM TEMPORALE/BROCA CONNECTIONS

The various specialized areas of the brain must be connected to each other, *e.g.* vision to speech, vision to movement, hearing to speech; this is achieved through the long and short association fibres connecting areas within the same hemisphere, and the corpus callosum and anterior and posterior commissures connecting areas between the two cerebral hemispheres. These connections form after birth and account for the development of certain skills (Fig. 1.6).

Wernicke's area is connected by long intracortical (within the same hemisphere) and intercortical (connection to opposite hemisphere) association fibres that can be readily demonstrated on dissection of the brain (Fig. 1.7). The most prominent are those that form the arcuate fasciculus: this connects Wernicke's area to Broca's motor speech area in the left third frontal convolution. It is through this direct connection that once a word or phrase is heard, discriminated and memorized, it can be sent directly to the motor output without any cognitive understanding. Such rote memory of words and phrases allows 'cocktail party' type conversation as well as repeating what is said as an echo (echolalia). This ability

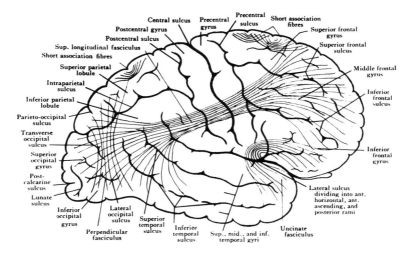

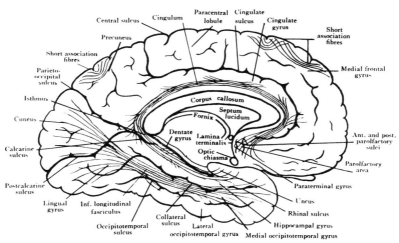

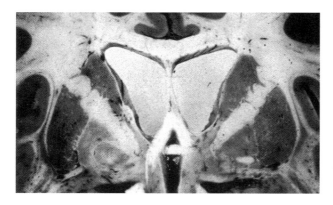

Fig. 1.6. *(Above)* Diagrammatic representations of the fibre tracts in the white matter connecting the various parts of the same cerebral hemisphere together.

(Left) Brain section showing the fibre tracts of white matter joining the two cerebral hemispheres, *i.e.* corpus callosum and anterior commissure.

13

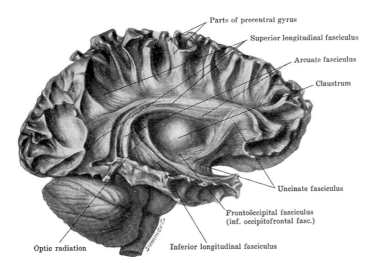

Parts of precentral gyrus

Superior longitudinal fasciculus

Arcuate fasciculus

Claustrum

Uncinate fasciculus

Frontoöccipital fasciculus
(inf. occipitofrontal fasc.)

Optic radiation

Inferior longitudinal fasciculus

Fig. 1.7. Cut-away section of brain with the cerebral grey matter removed, showing that although the white matter appears homogeneous it is in reality a mass of 'cables' joining the various parts of the brain. The arcuate fasciculus joining Broca's and Wernicke's areas can be seen as a large bundle arching over the basal ganglia. (Reproduced by permission from Last 1956.)

is also preserved as sentence repetition in transcortical aphasia. The interconnection of Broca's and Wernicke's areas is the basis of the so-called Wernicke–Geschwind model of human speech and explains the various forms of aphasia. It is necessary to have a two-way 'to and fro' connection between Broca's and Wernicke's areas so that we can plan a reply linked to the word store (lexicon) (see later).

TRANSCORTICAL APHASIAS

If the arcuate fibres are interrupted then the sensory and motor aspects of speech would be expected to be separated and independent. This gives rise in the verbal child to what has been described as transcortical aphasia and is usually divided into a transcortical motor and a transcortical sensory aphasia. The important feature about this group of speech and language disorders is that there is retention of the ability to repeat a sentence that the child does not understand. Transcortical sensory aphasia is like classical sensory aphasia: there is inability to understand what is said, but spontaneous or echoed speech is well pronounced.

Section 1.4—Localization of memories
ANATOMY AND LOCALIZATION

Does the brain store learned memories in localized areas? If we believe that the brain is the organ of learning and that memories are stored, in a physical sense, similar to any other computer then it cannot be in a vague generalized way in a mass of jelly as the black box approach to holistic psychology suggests. Any computer disk must be formatted to arrange the memories in a retrievable form at specified addresses. The localization of permanently

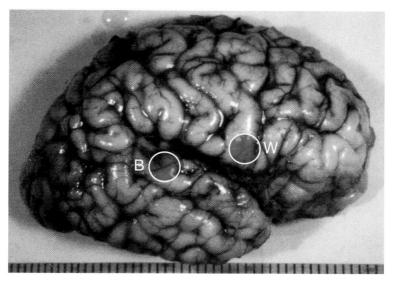

Fig. 1.8. Lateral view of the brain showing that superficially Broca's area (B) and Wernicke's area (W) appear distant and separate due to the sylvian fissure.

stored data in the cerebral cortex is in reality the equivalent of the brain's hard disk: it is formatted so that specific addresses (*i.e.* localities in the brain) are committed to specific learning modalities.

The history of ideas on localization is interesting. It was Auburtin (1825–1893) whose gruesome experiment started the search for localization. He had a patient who in attempting suicide blew off the front of his skull. Auburtin showed that by pressing on his exposed frontal lobes with a spatula he could arrest the patient's speech. He subsequently worked with Broca to show that it was expression, not comprehension of speech, that was situated in the frontal region on the left side (Fig. 1.8). Broca (1865), in describing the brain of his original aphasic patient, noted a large lesion encompassing the left insula and frontal, central and parietal operculum. He attributed this patient's aphasia to involvement of the frontal operculum, and tended to ignore the overall extent of the lesion. Gall, a phrenologist, noted that talkative people had large eyes, and assumed the eyes to have become prominent by displacement from hypertrophy of nearby orbital regions of the overlying brain (see Head 1926). Wernicke showed that aphasia with comprehension loss was due to left-sided lesions, and Dejerine completed the language dominance theory of the left hemisphere by showing that reading and writing skills were also dependent upon an intact left cerebral hemisphere. Subsequently, Penfield and Roberts (1959) studied the effects of stimulating the exposed brain of conscious patients during neurosurgery, demonstrating the hearing of buzzing from the auditory area, flashing light sensation from the visual area and simple movements from the motor area, but complex more organized sensations from the temporal lobes. Luria (1966) looked in particular at the effects on speech of localized gunshot wounds. These

TABLE 1.2
Methods for the study of the localization
of learning

Anatomical structure—hard wiring
Pathological and surgical lesions
Electrical stimulation—Penfield
Electroencephalography—brain mapping
Indwelling electrodes
Evoked potentials
Dichotic listening
CT of lesions
MRI of lesions
PET
Functional MRI
Wada testing
Split brain studies

studies are now of historical interest only, since with modern MRI, SPECT, PET and now functional MRI we can look at normal people with no pathology and also study in fine detail pathology known to be strictly localized (Table 1.2).

HARD-WIRING

In classical clinical neurology, when deducing areas of specialization in the cerebral cortex from the study of patients with localized pathology, one always had the anxiety that hypoxia, ischaemia or the effects of raised intracranial pressure could be diffuse, not confined to the immediate area of disease, even with a circumscribed lesion such as a contusion, tumour or infarct. These historical studies have not, on the whole, been proved to be wrong. The cerebral cortex shows a pattern of gyri and sulci that allows certain landmarks such as the central sulcus and motor strip, the calcarine cortex for vision and Heschl's gyrus for hearing to be easily identified. These may be grossly distorted in hydrocephalus, yet function is normal, so that surface anatomy is unreliable. As a result of histological studies, Brodman (1909) showed that the cortex could be divided into defined areas to which he gave numbers: the Brodman map (Fig. 1.9). Although this remained a largely academic tool, it is now becoming important as we need to accurately define the area of cortex that we are demonstrating with functional studies.

All this work suggested the anatomical localization of motor speech was in the inferior motor strip, *i.e.* Broca's area. The localization of vision is in the occipital area (Brodman area 17), motor skills in the precentral gyrus (Brodman area 4), somatic sensation in the posterior central gyrus (Brodman area 1) and hearing in the superior temporal Heschl's gyrus (Brodman area 41). These all represent the primary motor and perceptual areas.

These primary 'hard-wired' areas are committed to the function dictated by the anatomy and cannot be replaced if damaged. They are not 'plastic' but represent only 5 per cent of the total area of cerebral cortex. Primary areas are the areas damaged in cortical blindness, cerebral palsy and cortical deafness. The premotor area is wired to the pyramidal tract, the calcarine cortex to the optic tract, Heschl's gyrus to the auditory lemniscal system, and sensory

16

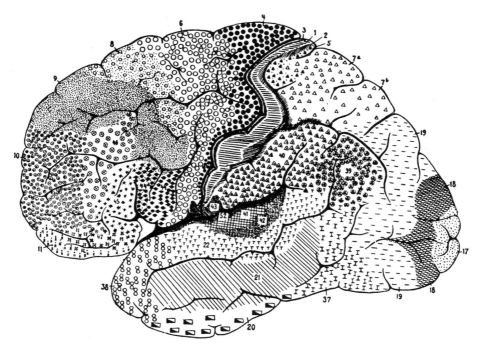

Fig. 1.9. Brodman's map of the histological appearance of the cerebral cortex, showing that that like the white matter it is not a homogeneous mass but varies from area to area with the predetermined function. Note that even areas 41 and 42, Wernicke's area, are different in cellular structure. These areas can now be delineated by functional studies.

fibres from the thalamus to the postcentral gyrus. The same hard-wired anatomical pathway has already been described from cochlea to Heschl's gyrus and then to Broca's area. The lips, tongue and palate, which are very important for speech and learned oral skills, have a high neuron density and big somatotopic representation in the premotor area. These areas then send their messages by part of the pyramidal tract known as the corticobulbar pathway, and this descends to the brainstem to synapse on the brainstem nuclei such as the nucleus ambiguus, nucleus solitarius and the vagal motor nucleus to control the muscles of speech, mastication and swallowing, described later.

ASSOCIATION AREAS
Adjacent to each primary area is an association area where material from perception, *i.e.* vision, hearing, tactile or motor planning, is stored. Using modern techniques of functional imaging one can show that motor planning occurs in the motor association area, execution in the precentral gyrus, and sequencing in the supplementary motor area. Speaking can be shown to be associated with the association area for lips, tongue and palate (Broca) and writing with the association area for the hand (graphomotor centre).

17

TABLE 1.3
Functions of the right and left hemispheres of the brain

Right cerebral hemisphere	Left cerebral hemisphere
Visual recognition faces, shapes	Word recognition
Colour, objects—pictographs	
Space, shape direction (visuospatial)	Understanding—concepts
	Reading
Drawing	Writing
	Spelling
Constructional praxis	Speech
	Facial expression
Gesture recognition	
Manipulo/spatial (visuomotor)	Verbal reasoning
Arithmetic, number	
Musical appreciation	
Intonational pattern imposed upon speech—singing	
Flight	Fight
Gestalt function	

Reading depends upon the visual association area on the left (Table 1.3), *i.e.* it is involved in the recognition of visual symbols that have a linguistic meaning. This may not be the case in Chinese pictography where the symbol does not relate to a phonological equivalent. The integration of phonological awareness of heard speech with the graphemes of written speech requires the angular gyrus. The written word so analysed is still 'inwardly heard' in Wernicke's area. The same language areas of the planum temporale, *i.e.* Wernicke's area, also light up when lip-reading. Deaf people lose the ability to understand sign language after left hemisphere lesions.

Visual recognition of objects, discrimination of faces, shapes and geometrical forms, colour recognition and naming, and sense of direction (*i.e.* cognitive maps) all depend upon the visual association area of the right hemisphere. It is thought that we develop a visual lexicon in the same way as a verbal one: we have a dictionary of pictographs as to what represents a basic chair, table, face, house, etc. The visual association areas on the right can be shown to 'light up' differentially when looking at scenes or faces compared to language-based materials. As definition of imaging improves one can show that discrete areas of visual cerebral cortex are committed to processing for faces, geometrical forms, central colour vision, speed of movement and written words, and that each of these abilities can be lost in isolation. Naming objects by shape, colour, number or position requires a visual perception in the right hemisphere to be linked by the corpus callosum and angular gyrus with the lexicon on the left and so can be vulnerable to disruption. Counting is also initially based upon visual perception of multiple 'concrete' objects, such as counting blocks and fingers, and so is right-hemisphere dependent. Later a written symbol system or language allows us to internalize number concepts, *i.e.* mental arithmetic.

This localization within the cerebral cortex means that the shape, size, colour, texture, temperature, smell, taste, and phonemic (pronunciation) and graphemic (written) structure, as well as biographical details of an object, are all stored in different areas of the brain and on different sides.

CEREBRAL DOMINANCE

It is thought that the very young infant uses both sides of the brain with a mirror pattern of learning for each modality—speech, reading, shape copying, drawing, writing and postural movement—so which mirror image appears it may be a chance occurrence. The more *learned* a skill, *e.g.* speech or hand manipulation, the more it needs to be lateralized to one side of the brain. The more midline an ability, *e.g.* biting, chewing, swallowing, bladder and bowel control, the less it is lateralized, thus either hemisphere will sustain the function, and the ability persists after hemispherectomy. This is why speech can be lost but bite, chew and swallow are preserved. In the absence of a corpus callosum, the cerebral hemispheres continue to act as two separate brains with the memories from one entering consciousness without reference to the other hemisphere.

If the infantile pattern of bilateral learning persisted then mirror interference would be a constant problem, especially where direction was important. The child would exhibit (a) reversal on copying shapes, (b) reversal with patterns, *e.g.* block design, (c) right/left confusion on self or mannequin, (d) difficulty with imitation of gestures, (e) finger agnosia, (f) dysgraphaesthesia, (g) mirror movements to opposite side, (h) mirror posture on the Fog test, (i) speech reversals involving sound, word or phrase, (j) reading reversals such as *was/saw*, *god/dog*, and (k) writing reversals of letters (*b/d*, *m/n*) or words (*no/on*).

In order to prevent this interference and confusion continuing there must be suppression of one directional pattern in favour of the other: learning becomes localized to one side of the brain, in one place, with inhibition of the opposite side through the corpus callosum (reciprocal cerebral inhibition). This is what is meant by the acquisition of dominance that tends to occur between 3 and 7 years. Acquisition of dominance is under genetic control, showing variability, and so will follow a normal distribution curve with a mean around 5 years at school entry. One would therefore expect 3 per cent of children (*i.e.* those below the third centile) to be very slow in the acquisition of dominance. There are some families in which dominance is acquired even more slowly. This will be more obvious in boys than in girls because the brain always develops more slowly in boys, and the left hemisphere more slowly than the right. Some children do not achieve this until well into the school years, and the occasional child never achieves complete dominance.

If a 3-year-old who is developing speech predominantly in the left hemisphere suffers damage to the speech areas on that side, then after a period of mutism, dysphasia, confusion and reversals s/he will learn to speak completely normally using the opposite hemisphere. At age 10 years this recovery would not be possible. It is claimed that 100 per cent of children with an acquired left unilateral lesion will recover from aphasia (Byers and McLean 1962). Over 70 per cent of congenital hemiplegia cases are right-sided, *i.e.* left-brain infarcts, but aphasia is rare, although 40 per cent of affected children may be slower in speaking. Proof that speech has been transferred to the right hemisphere is shown when hemispherectomy is used to control epilepsy arising in the damaged side. Removal of the abnormal hemisphere, *i.e.* the left one, does not result in any deterioration in speech, which may in fact improve with control of the associated epilepsy (Basser 1962).

Section 1.5—Cognition: concept formation and understanding

Cognition derives from the Latin *cognitio*, meaning knowledge or understanding. With the development of understanding we are able to say, "I know", that is, I have knowledge, I possess a collection of acquired data on that subject, I can group and bring together all this information into short-term memory and consciousness. This forms a *concept* so that I can say that I understand, for example, what is meant by an orange and I can define it.

If we take the concept of an orange, then the phonetic sound sequence, smell, taste, colour, size, texture, and written spelling (graphemic sequence), together with facts such as that it is a citrus fruit, it contains vitamin C, there are Jaffas and blood oranges, and they come from Israel, Spain, etc., are, as discussed above, all learned memories stored in different parts of the brain. Each of these memories by itself is not of any great use, and would be very difficult to access, unless a form of logical computer programme were to go through every stored memory in the brain each time we saw, heard, smelled, tasted or felt anything. The time when a particular memory component of a concept was initially laid down from first perception may differ from a recent memory by 50 or more years, and it would be extremely inefficient if a whole lifetime of individual memories had to be gone through sequentially to extract one fact. The human brain is not *logical* like an ordinary computer, which runs through all its information in a preset mathematical order dictated by the software, but is *associative*, scanning all memories in the whole cerebral cortex at the same time in response to the trigger word or symbol looking for relevant data to 'light up'. These individual memories are then all brought into short-term memory and so into consciousness. It follows that what tie together data on a common theme, allowing items to be selected from the mass of other data in each part of the brain, are the systems of symbols that form languages.

These spoken or written word, numerical, chemical, geometric or electronic symbols, visual images, smells or tastes trigger all memories relevant to the stimulus so that all these components together form a *concept*. The concept once formed can be entered by any individual memory component, *e.g.* the smell or taste of an orange, as well as its appearance or name. The individual memories are retrieved from all the different addresses in the cerebral cortex and brought together into short-term memory (the capacity of consciousness), and so into conscious thought (thought being defined as the current content of consciousness). One *re-cognizes* the object and is able to say, "I understand what that is", "I have previous knowledge." If an orange were square, blue in colour, or tasted like a peach, the incongruity compared to the existing concept would cause us to recognize that this was discordant and make us unsure whether we understood what it was. One does not therefore need to take sides as a language localizer versus a believer in holistic whole brain function: words, *i.e.* the lexicon, are localized, but inner language as defined by understanding or comprehension requires all parts of the brain.

SHORT-TERM MEMORY

Long-term permanent memories are stored in the cerebral cortex, which is the brain's hard disk and is formatted in the sense that memories are stored in a particular place, *i.e.* address. Short-term memory is the equivalent of RAM (random access memory) in computer terms. It is not permanent, is easily removed, and so probably is due to oscillating circuits in the reticular formation. Just as a whole morning's work on a computer, if left in RAM and not saved to hard disk, is lost if the computer is switched off, so our current thoughts in short-term memory go with distraction, sleep or anaesthesia. The saving of our thoughts from perception or reasoning currently in short-term memory into the permanent memory of the cerebral cortex is by the equivalent of a 'save command' in the anterior temporal lobe. If this is damaged by disease or surgery no new memories can be stored (Brown and Minns 1999).

Just as all processing in a computer must be done in RAM after retrieval from hard disk and external sources, so all recognition, understanding and reasoning can only occur if perception from the senses and memories from the cerebral cortex are brought back into short-term memory. It is only then that they become conscious. Short-term memory is in effect the capacity of consciousness, and in our computer analogy is the equivalent of what is on the VDU screen.

Thoughts can be processed or computed by *verbal reasoning*. Verbal reasoning consists of comparing each component of the concept: for instance, if asked, "What is the difference between an orange and an apple?" we would compare size, shape, colour, taste and smell to see if they were similar or different. As a result of this reasoning, we can come to a *decision*: they are similar or different. We can compare an apple with an orange (an easy process), socialism with communism (a narrow concept), or the substantia nigra with the locus coeruleus (a barely existing concept, so understanding is limited). One must have multiple stored facts, *i.e.* knowledge on a subject, in order to form a concept. The more individual memories there are, *i.e.* the more components to the concept, the greater the depth of understanding. In the mature adult these may not be solely dependent upon perception but can be abstract concepts, *e.g.* feminism, 'the Holy Spirit'.

These mental abilities or processes of *perception, recognition, understanding, verbal reasoning* and *decision making* are the basis of the mind and what we attempt to test in intelligence tests.

Section 1.6—Symbolic function and inner language

The way in which memories acquired at different times in our lives and stored in different parts of the brain are classified into concepts depends upon a structured symbol system, which we call a language. A language therefore is a system of symbols that we use to classify and code data stored in different places in the cerebral cortex but on a common theme. Although this language is usually based upon words (spoken and written), other symbol systems such as chemical symbols, electronic circuitry, musical notation, algebraic and arithmetic symbols are also languages allowing memories to be grouped into concepts and so facilitating understanding and reasoning. A chemist can think in terms of benzene rings and can reason what happens if s/he places an hydroxyl group on a steroid nucleus at a certain point. The electronics engineer can think in terms of oscillator circuits. Musically stimulated people show an increase in cerebral blood flow to the right non-dominant temporal area, but a musically literate person shows bilateral response, *i.e.* processing music as a language. Deaf children using sign language will also activate language receptive areas in the left temporal lobe. It is interesting that deaf children will talk to themselves in sign language, and deaf–blind children taught a digital language can be seen translating Braille felt with one hand into digital language with the other, so one must not be restrictive and think only of spoken words as the language. As described above, we have a spatial vocabulary or lexicon of simple outline shapes or pictographs that allows us to recognize, for instance, all faces, chairs or houses as having certain basic common features upon which the concept can then be built. Chinese people who speak Cantonese and read Mandarin (a pictographic written form), and hence have no spelling of the word, show that words and their spatial representation need not be the same or depend upon phonetic analysis with a strict grapheme-to-phoneme association.

Limited ability to use a symbol system in order to create concepts and so create understanding and verbal reasoning is the basic defect in learning disability. In learning disability, the abilities of the brain necessary for language, memory recall, thought and reasoning are impaired. Thus, learning disability is global delay in the development of cognitive learning in order to differentiate it from the specific learning disorders—dysphasia, dysgraphia, dyscalculia, dyslexia and dyspraxia (Brown and Minns 1999).

A distinction is drawn between learning with understanding and rote or memory learning without understanding. It is also necessary to differentiate other non-cognitive learning, such as learning to sit, crawl and walk, which really depend upon the stage of brain maturation. Motor learning is not cognitive, does not depend upon a language or symbol system, uses different brain circuits, and can be lost or maintained independent of cognitive function.

INTELLIGENCE

Although most people when asked to define learning disability would include a low IQ in the definition, they would have much more difficulty if then asked to define intelligence. Is it general ability, common sense, what intelligence tests test, or native wit (Wechsler 1945); and then, what do intelligence tests test? At the end of the 19th century, Binet in Paris was asked to devise some method of testing children to sort out those who would benefit from schooling. He devised a series of graded test items to assess range of abilities in language, drawing, spatial concepts, numeracy, hand skills, etc., and this formed the basis of the Stanford–Binet Intelligence Scale. Language ability plays a very important part in all IQ tests of general ability, and a vocabulary test and verbal reasoning play a major role. If one were to choose a single subtest to predict later abilities in reading, writing and spelling, then a test of active vocabulary would be first choice.

These tests were carried out on large numbers of children to establish what the normal child should be able to do at different ages. Standardized tests could then establish the mental age of a patient; compared with the chronological age and expressed as a percentage this gives an intelligence quotient, as:

$$IQ = \frac{\text{Mental age} \times 100}{\text{Chronological age}}$$

Several points of importance emerge from this. First, it is the intelligence quotient that is constant and not intelligence: intelligence increases with age and is a function of a child's brain development and life experience. Second, intelligence is not a static innate function of the individual but is dependent upon genetic factors and the environment in which the child has been reared, as well as upon the integrity of the sensory mechanisms through which stimuli from the environment can reach her/him.

RECEPTIVE APHASIA (DEVELOPMENTAL SEMANTIC DYSPHASIA, SEMANTIC–PRAGMATIC DISORDER, SPECIFIC LANGUAGE IMPAIRMENT, SEVERE FORM OF DEVELOPMENTAL SPEECH RETARDATION SYNDROME)

The above heading illustrates the difficulty with nomenclature in the whole field of paediatric aphasiology: clinical neurologists, psychologists, psycholinguists and speech therapists all use their own terminology, and worse still, this changes with fashion. Children vary from adults, and developmental disorders in children differ from acquired diseases. In the UK, specific language impairment (SLI) has tended to become a blanket term for all developmental speech and language disorders, while dysphasia is retained in the USA. There are, of course, examples of pure specific developmental disorders such as dyslexia, dysgraphia, dysmusia and dyscalculia, as well as pure phonological delay (dyslalia) and pure receptive aphasia. In the severe form of developmental speech disorder all aspects of speech—phonological, syntactical, pragmatic, prosodic and semantic—are affected. The autistic spectrum disorder with speech delay, developmental semantic disorder and gross disturbance of nonverbal communication illustrates the impurity of many developmental speech syndromes. Certain causes of learning disorder such as Klinefelter syndrome, fragile X syndrome and Angelman syndrome may have much more profound involvement of language than of other cognitive learning abilities.

It is estimated that 8 per cent of boys and 6 per cent of girls have a developmental language impairment. Pure cases of developmental receptive dysphasia are usually genetic with dominant inheritance, and about one-third (30–46 per cent) have a positive history in a first-degree relative (Bishop *et al.* 1995). Adoption or twin studies suggest that genetic factors are more important than environmental ones. Subsequent slow development of higher language functions, affecting reading, writing and spelling, is common, affecting 50 per cent of children. This means that school performance as well as future job prospects will be poorer than expected in children with genetic language impairment syndromes. There may be a history of dyslexia in other members of the family, and not necessarily receptive aphasia. The ability to repeat nonsense words is markedly impaired in children and adults who may appear to have 'grown out' of the condition. This test is now used to select out siblings or even adults with the genetic trend, and this is making study of the clinical genetics much easier, so that pure cohorts can be obtained for study at the molecular genetics level.

Like all developmental disorders, it may be more severe in the male. Children with congenital, presumed genetic dysphasia have normal imaging with no demonstrable pathological legions; they do not show increased blood flow to the left hemisphere during dichotic stimulation compared to normal controls (Chiron *et al.* 1999). They show hypoperfusion in the left temporoparietal region on SPECT (Denays *et al.* 1989).

Semantic receptive dysphasia of childhood, including central deafness, constitutes a profound disorder of inner language, *i.e.* the ability to use words to form concepts in order to understand, think and reason (see above). The child does not understand the simplest of commands and may have little or no spoken speech before 3 years. S/he loves music and obviously is able to hear and can discriminate and remember a sequence of tones of varying pitch but not sound sequences that have a linguistic meaning. Songs may be sung with true sense of tune, rhythm and pitch. Ability to comprehend language through a visual mode is preserved. This may lead to the 'video addict syndrome': the child will sit for hours watching videos, which they memorize nearly frame for frame by the pictures, but cannot understand the sound. They may watch foreign-language TV programmes, ignoring the sound. They often develop a good passive vocabulary for things that have a visual rather than a linguistic representation, *e.g.* objects, pictures, or things seen on TV or video, so that the child will perform better on tests of passive vocabulary that require identification of pictures by name such as the English Picture Vocabulary or Peabody Picture Vocabulary scales. The child may fail to understand simple commands to bring an object when there is no visual cue. The parents often subconsciously use a lot of gesture to reinforce their speech to the child. Active vocabulary is very poor and retarded. In pure cases, speech may be preserved on repetition of prelearned phrases, with accurate phonological development; these children may superficially appear to be 'chatty' and articulate, but closer inspection of their language reveals echolalia, perseverations, circumlocutions and semantic paraphrasias and errors. In most cases, speech is also delayed, especially with associated word deafness. Their comprehension is always delayed compared to their expression, and they fail to understand their own speech.

As development proceeds and improvement occurs they may be able to recognize and name objects but be unable to carry out more complex language tasks such as classifying or categorizing. They cannot cope with abstract notions such as time, *e.g. in a minute*, *today*, *yesterday*, *now*, *later*. Symbolic and pretend play is delayed as the child cannot 'say to her/himself', which is necessary to sustain play with toy cars or doll's houses but not with nonverbalized play such as Lego or painting.

It can be difficult to differentiate these conditions from learning disability and autism, unless the child can be shown to have normal or advanced development in nonverbal spatial skills, *e.g.* formboards (which may be completed with astonishing rapidity), block design, matrices such as Raven's, mazes, drawing geometrical shapes or people, and completing jigsaws. A study of Table 1.3, showing the functions of the cerebral hemispheres, indicates that the difficulties all involve left-sided functions, while the strengths (music, object recognition, shape sense, hand skills) are all right-sided. Reading, which is a language skill, will be retarded; however, the good spatial memory means that a 'look and say' approach allows the child to remember words as shapes (the development of phonological awareness), although the ability to split words into individual sounds remains difficult.

Behaviour in the second year may show autistic features that usually resolve, but temper tantrums, screaming episodes and marked fight and flight response to minor frustrations may dominate the picture for the parents. The child is uncooperative during neurological examination or attempted psychological testing. The clinician may be struck by their bizarre behaviour and overlook their language disorder.

Their pragmatic use of language is impaired: they do not take turns in conversation or maintain a topic, and they do not understand the nature of sarcasm or the adjustments required in language depending on the other person, *e.g.* sibling compared to teacher. There is a sensation of tangential conversation and the impression that most of the work is being done by the listener when trying to establish a theme to the communication. In most cases there is marked improvement by school entry at age 5 years. Persistence beyond this age carries a more worrying prognosis.

If nonverbal communication is grossly disturbed, the disorder merges into autistic spectrum disorder or Asperger syndrome (Bishop and Rosenbloom 1987). Unfortunately, 'lumping' of diagnostic categories has resulted in children with no autistic features, in terms of a *nonverbal/emotional* communication disorder, also being diagnosed with autistic spectrum disorder. The increase in the number of children with a diagnosis of autism may therefore be due in part to a more decisive differentiation of specific language disorders from learning disorder and the inclusion of children previously considered dysphasic. This means that we cannot be sure if there is a real increase in incidence, and makes elucidation of aetiology, whether true or false (such as its relationship to immunization), impossible.

Differentiation of a pure developmental language disorder from autism or learning disability is very difficult. These complicated cases are typically mute or severely dysfluent, and if they do speak, their articulation is grossly defective. Such children show gross auditory inattention to speech, and clearly great care must be taken to exclude a peripheral high tone hearing loss, which is easier if musical ability and phrase repetition is preserved.

Acquired Receptive Dysphasia, Wernicke's Dysphasia, Central Aphasia
Damage to the dominant temporal lobe, in the posterior part of the superior temporal gyrus and the planum temporale, produces a receptive dysphasia. The aetiologies include head injury with extradural haematoma, direct contusional injury, contracoup injury or swirling of the brain against the edge of the sphenoidal wing, epileptic dysphasia, temporal lobe abscess from middle ear infection, emboli, cortical thrombophlebitis, herpes simplex encephalitis, meningitis and temporal lobe tumour.

In the adult a fluent aphasia (Wernicke's aphasia) results, with well-pronounced jargon speech and neologisms, whereas the clinical picture in childhood is dominated by mutism. As the mutism resolves, the comprehension difficulties persist and include the child's understanding of her/his own speech. In Wernicke's aphasia the loss of understanding of spoken speech can be total or affect only certain words and complex sentences: there is also loss of the ability to understand the written word. The wrong syntactical construction of sentences occurs, which may be made up of nonexistent words (neologisms). A word may get stuck and keep coming out in subsequent sentences, *i.e.* word perseveration. The patient is not aware of the problem, due to the comprehension difficulty, compared to a pure nominal aphasia that causes intense frustration. Reading skills are usually lost. Copying is preserved but spontaneous writing shows the same mistakes as in the spoken word.

Epileptic Dysphasia: The Landau–Kleffner Syndrome
Epileptic aphasia, along with post-traumatic aphasia, is the commonest acquired aphasia

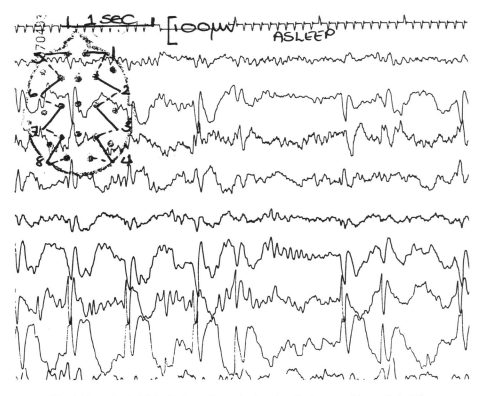

Fig. 1.10. EEG of child with loss of speech, showing discharges without clinical fits.

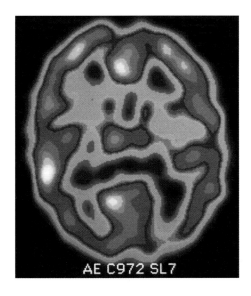

AE C972 SL7

Fig. 1.11. SPECT scan showing hypometabolic area focal to the left temporal lobe.

in children and more common than trauma as a cause of lasting aphasia. Onset is classically in the 3–5 year age group; it may start before 2 years, with autistic features rather than aphasia being most obvious, or occur after 7 years or very rarely in the adult. Fits may be polymorphic, *i.e.* tonic–clonic, partial or more often a complex absence. The fits are not always prominent and the epilepsy may not be considered severe. The loss of speech can be sudden or gradually evolve. CT and MRI are usually normal with no demonstrable encephalitis such as that due to herpes simplex virus or cortical dysplasia. The EEG is always epileptic but most characteristic is the presence of a continuous epileptic discharge (electrical status epilepticus) in slow (non-eye-movement) sleep (ESES). This may occupy 80 per cent of sleep. Auditory agnosia and a receptive dysphasia are the commonest speech disorder seen, but expressive dysphasia or mutism often become prominent in the Landau–Kleffner syndrome. In this disorder language regresses in association with EEG spike and wave activity in one or both temporal lobes, and the speech loss appears to parallel the EEG abnormality, particularly status in sleep, suggesting that the epileptic discharge is the prime cause (Fig. 1.10). It is thought that the clinical symptomatology results from disruption of auditory input into Wernicke's area. PET and SPECT most commonly show hypometabolic areas in one or both temporal lobes, and there may be reduced glucose metabolism in the superior temporal gyrus, *i.e.* Wernicke's area (Fig. 1.11) (O'Tuama *et al.* 1992, Guerreiro *et al.* 1996). The child may appear to 'switch off', losing social contact and nonverbal communication— that is, an acute onset of autistic behaviour; wild disruptive hyperkinetic behaviour is a prominent intractable symptom in some children. The speech abnormality will usually improve with treatment and time, but reading and spelling difficulty can persist for years. If the disorder has an onset before 4 years or is left untreated for a year, then over 60 per cent of cases may have long-term cognitive problems (Rossi *et al.* 1999). Treatment with steroids such as ACTH or benzodiazepines (clobazam or nitrazepam), after sensitivity to the drug has been demonstrated by intravenous administration during EEG monitoring, can reverse the aphasia.

The syndrome in its full form is relatively rare, although some authors report over 20 cases; deterioration of speech in children with epilepsy and a hypometabolic encephalopathy is more common (O'Regan *et al.* 1998). It is now thought that the common, genetically determined, 'benign rolandic epilepsy' (benign partial epilepsy) is one end of a spectrum with 'malignant rolandic epilepsy' at the other, being the same as Landau–Kleffner syndrome: all show sleep activation of the EEG (de Negri 1997).

Section 1.7—Nonverbal communication
Up to now we have considered verbal communication and understanding by the formation of concepts but there is another communication system intricately intertwined known as nonverbal communication. This system recognizes the person communicating as a fellow human being with emotion and feelings, which sets them apart from inanimate objects. We equally need to be able to receive the signals from the other person, interpret them with the accompanying feeling, and then signal back our emotional response. Emotional feelings are generated in the limbic system and reach consciousness by creating 'affect', *i.e.* feelings, such as empathy, love, hate, disbelief, boredom, anger, anxiety, happiness, ecstasy, sadness

and depression, which are superimposed on the thoughts occupying our consciousness and then communicated subconsciously back to the other person as intonation of voice, hand gesture and facial expression.

It is probable that emotional memories are stored in the cingulate gyrus on the right side and are expressed via the supplementary motor area to the extrapyramidal system. When an event or a memory is remembered and brought back into short-term memory then the emotion that accompanied that event is also remembered and 'felt', and this is why we enjoy reminiscences with old friends. We cannot conjure up happiness or joy unless we remember a previous event when we felt that emotion. Music is another way of bringing back emotional memories.

ANATOMY OF EMOTION

The anatomical basis of emotion was suggested by Papez (1937) and thought to consist of the medial temporal lobe structures the hypothalamus, amygdala and hippocampus, together with the limbic system and cingulate gyrus of the nondominant right cerebral hemisphere. The hypothalamus is well known to be responsible for sexual maturation, thirst, hunger, sleep, rage and stress reactions. The hippocampus runs along the medial side of the temporal lobe and the cingulate gyrus along the medial side of the cerebral hemispheres, and is really a continuous band in the shape of a letter C. It is this C which is the 'limbic system', so called by Broca (1878) because it resembled a band or fringe. It was thought by Broca to be the brutal or animal brain, the palaeomammalian brain, and in animals is related to smell and innate behaviours. It represents the oldest part of the cerebral cortex, the archicortex, and has another outer band (like an annual ring of a tree) of limbic mesocortex and then a further outer ring, the limbic neocortex. The amygdalar division of the archicortex serves the oldest functions, for self-preservation, *i.e.* fight or flight, feeding and drinking. The middle septal division has to do with social mating, procreation and sex. The outer limbic neocortex (thalamocingulate) is to do with maternal behaviour, separation anxiety and play (Maclean 1992). This means that certain behaviours to do with feeding and self-preservation and then procreation and care of the young are preprogrammed in the older parts of the emotional brain as a kind of computer ROM (read-only memory). Crying and laughter are also thought to depend upon these brain circuits.

The barking of dogs, chirping of birds, mooing of cows and the specific cries of a human neonate (birth cry, hunger cry, pain cry) are not languages as claimed by Charles Darwin. They are certainly a definite form of communication but relate more to the innate emotional behaviour patterns described above. The language of the limbic/extrapyramidal system signifies hunger, pain, danger, anger or invasion of territory.

In the more mature person there may be an emotional vocabulary used to indicate feelings rather than thoughts. Swear words and expletives ("Damn!", "Jesus Christ!", "Oh shit!") come out automatically when one is frustrated, even in an inappropriate place, and are thought to represent separate emotional language that can be preserved in aphasia. Smith (1972) showed that, even after a total left hemispherectomy for tumour, not only could his patient swear, but he could also sing hymn tunes with words even though aphasic. An aphasic patient may not be able to repeat the word 'goodbye' and yet says it spontaneously when a friend leaves. Emotional swearing and expletives dominate the picture in Tourette syndrome.

RECEPTIVE DYSPROSODIA

We speak words expressing the thoughts in our left hemisphere but we express the emotions from the right hemisphere about how we feel through the nonverbal communication that is superimposed upon this verbal communication (George *et al.* 1996). Failure to be able to interpret these emotional signals forms a receptive dysprosodia and is seen in right hemisphere dysfunction (Cohen *et al.* 1994) and is a core problem in autism. If a child cannot appreciate these signals of emotional feelings, then s/he does not know if a person is sad, upset with her/his behaviour or happy, and does not recognize the personal space of others.

Emotional cues are perceived through all five senses:

- *Auditory:* intonation of voice and music are recognized by the same area, *i.e.* the planum temporale of the right cerebral hemisphere
- *Visual:* appreciation of beauty/ugliness, facial recognition, and recognition of facial expression as in anger, happiness or sadness are by the right visual association area; sustained eye-to-eye contact and pupillary changes denote sexual interest
- *Tactile:* erogenous zones, stroke, caress
- *Olfactory:* food, excreta, perfume, body odour, pheromones
- *Taste:* food, wine.

There is no point in looking a person in the eye, if one cannot interpret the emotional signals: one therefore lacks orientation to nonverbal cues. The child may not see any difference between people and objects (sits on a knee as if a chair, holds a face as if a ball). Because of an inability to decode emotional information the child may appear detached. S/he may not 'greet' a parent or come for comfort if hurt; s/he does not use pretend play (mummies and daddies, doctors and nurses) and has no imagination with toys; s/he is a loner and does not interact with other children; s/he does not involve parents or adults in play by showing them books or toys.

EXPRESSIVE DYSPROSODIA

The expression of emotion is a motor act and includes hand gesture, sprightly gait, dilatation of pupils, periorbital muscles changing the size of the palpebral fissures, and facial muscle activity as with laughing, smiling and frowning. The larynx superimposes stress, pauses, and changes in pitch, volume and intonation upon the motor learned pattern of speech. Singing shows how words and music (*i.e.* intonation) can be united or separated. Broca's original aphasic patient could sing a melody without any difficulty. The right hemisphere controls musical tone recognition, pitch, rhythm and tune memory. We sing as we speak, and the intonation pattern accompanying speech can be likened to us constantly singing to a Gregorian chant (see above).

It is thought that emotional motor activity is expressed via the extrapyramidal system through the basal ganglia, and emotional expressive difficulties, *i.e.* an expressive dysprosodia, may occur in extrapyramidal disease when there may be inappropriate emotional expression. One may laugh at sad events or show sudden emotional incontinence with crying, shouting, laughing, anger or aggression that is not in context of environmental events. This can be seen in Sydenham's chorea (maniacal chorea) and juvenile Huntingdon's chorea. The child with hyperkinetic cerebral palsy may present with seemingly inappropriate facial expressions such as smile-like grimacing when distressed. The man with parkinsonism with bradykinesia, poor hand gesture from bradykinesia and rigidity, facial immobility and a monotonous voice with little change in tone or inflection appears to be sad and miserable even though he may not feel that way; he is interpreted as such by observers and this reinforces the situation. The speed of speech, writing and walking is also controlled by the same system, and cadences may be faster when happy and slower when sad.

In the same way that a child with receptive language disorder will show a secondary speech abnormality, the child with a developmental receptive dysprosodia (*i.e.* autism) cannot show normal emotional output and has not learned an emotional vocabulary. Most children with a receptive and expressive dysprosodia have in addition a disorder of inner language and spoken speech, *i.e.* it accompanies a receptive aphasia, producing a pervasive or total communication failure. This could have its origin in dysplasia of both temporal planes. A large majority of autistic children also have learning disability, most likely due to the aetiology affecting widespread areas of the brain as with tuberous sclerosis, West syndrome and chromosome disorders such as fragile X. Some children with an isolated severe receptive dysprosodia are intellectually normal with no receptive aphasia, *i.e.* have pure Kanner-type autism or Asperger syndrome.

REFERENCES

Abraham, S.S., Wallace, I.F., Gravel, J.S. (1996) 'Early otitis media and phonological development at age 2 years.' *Laryngoscope*, **106**, 727–732.
Anderson, B., Southern, B.D., Powers, R.E. (1999) 'Anatomic asymmetries of the superior temporal lobes: a post-mortem study.' *Neuropsychiatry, Neuropsychology and Behavioural Neurology*, **12**, 247–254.
Basser, L.S. (1962) 'Hemiplegia of early onset and the faculty of speech with special reference to the effect of hemispherectomy.' *Brain*, **85**, 427–460.
Bishop, D., Rosenbloom, L. (1987) 'Childhood language disorders: classification and overview.' *In:* Rutter, M., Yule, W. (Eds.) *Language Development and Disorders. Clinics in Developmental Medicine No. 101/102.* London: Mac Keith Press, pp. 16–41.
—— North, T., Doulen, C. (1995) 'Genetic basis of specific language impairment: evidence from a twin study.' *Developmental Medicine and Child Neurology*, **37**, 56–71.
Blakemore, C. (1974) 'Development of the mammalian visual systems.' *British Medical Bulletin*, 30, 152–157.
Brain, R. (1961) *Speech Disorders.* London: Butterworths.
Broca, P. (1865) 'Perte de parole. Ramollissement chronique et destruction partielle du lobe anterior gauche du cerveaux.' *Bulletin de la Société Anthropologique de Paris*, **2**, 219–229.
—— (1878) 'Anatomie comparée des circumvolution cérébrales. Le grand lobe limbique et la scissure limbique dans la cerie des mammifères.' *Revue Anthropologique*, **1**, 385–498.
Brodmann, K. (1909) *Vergleichende Lokalisationslehre der Grosshirnrinde.* Leipzig: Barth.
Brown, J.K., Minns, R. (1999) 'The neurological basis of learning disorders in children.' *In:* Whitmore, K., Hart, H., Willems, G. (Eds.) *A Neurodevelopmental Approach to Specific Learning Disorders. Clinics in Developmental Medicine No. 145.* London: Mac Keith Press, pp. 24–75.
Byers, R.K., McLean, W.T. (1962) 'Etiology and course of certain hemiplegias with aphasia in childhood.' *Pediatrics*, **29**, 376–383.
Chiron, C., Pinton, F., Maseure, M.C., Duvelleroy-Hormet, C., Leon, F., Billard, C. (1999) 'Hemispheric specialization using SPECT and stimulation tasks in children with dysphasia and dystrophia.' *Developmental Medicine and Child Neurology*, **41**, 512–520.

Chomsky, N. (1972) *Language and the Mind.* New York: Harcourt Brace Jovanovich.

Cohen, M.J., Branch, W.B., Hynd, G.W. (1994) 'Receptive prosody in children with left or right hemisphere dysfunction.' *Brain and Language,* **7,** 171–181.

Coucke, P., Van Camp, G., Djoyodiharjo, B., Smith, S.D., Frants, R.R., Padberg, G.W., Darby, J.K., Huizing, E.H., Cremers, C.W., Kimberling, W.J. (1994) 'Linkage of autosomal dominant hearing loss to the short arm of chromosome 1 in two families.' *New England Journal of Medicine,* **331,** 425–431.

Denays, R., Tondeur, M., Foulon, M., Verstraeten, F., Ham, H., Piepsz, A., Noel, P. (1989) 'Regional brain blood flow in congenital dysphasia: studies with technetium 99m HMPAO SPECT.' *Journal of Nuclear Medicine,* **30,** 1825–1829.

de Negri M. (1980) 'Electrical status epilepticus during sleep (ESES). Different clinical syndromes: towards a unifying view?' *Brain and Development,* **19,** 447–451.

Everett, N.B. (1965) *Functional Neuroanatomy.* London: Henry Kimpton.

Galaburda, A.M. (1993) 'Neuroanatomical basis of developmental dyslexia.' *Current Opinion in Neurobiology,* **11,** 161–173.

George, M.S., Purekh, P.I., Rosinsky, N., Ketter, T.A., Kimbrell, T.A., Heilman, K.M., Herscovitch, P. (1996) 'Understanding emotional prosody activates the right hemisphere regions.' *Archives of Neurology,* **53,** 665–670.

Geschwind, N., Levitsky, W. (1968) 'Human brain left–right asymmetries in temporal speech region.' *Science,* **161,** 186–187.

Ghazala, Q.R. (1993) 'Incantors – Circuit-bending and living instruments.' *Experimental Musical Instruments,* **8** (6), 18–21.

Guerreiro, M.M., Camargo, E.E., Kato, M. (1996) 'Brain single photon emission computed tomography imaging in Landau–Kleffner syndrome.' *Epilepsia,* **37,** 60–67.

Head, H. (1926) *Aphasia and Kindred Disorders of Speech.* London: Cambridge University Press.

Ingram, T.T.S. (1959) 'Specific developmental disorders of speech in childhood.' *Brain,* **82,** 446–450.

Johkura, K., Matsumoto, S., Hasegawa, O., Kuroiwa, Y. (1998) 'Defective auditory recognition after small haemorrhage in the inferior colliculi.' *Journal of the Neurological Sciences,* **161,** 91–96.

Kaga, M. (1999) 'Language disorders in Landau–Kleffner syndrome.' *Journal of Child Neurology,* **14,** 118–122.

Last, R.J. (1956) *Anatomy, Regional and Applied.* London: J. & A. Churchill.

Law, J., Conway, J. (1992) 'Effect of abuse and neglect on the development of children's speech and language.' *Developmental Medicine and Child Neurology,* **34,** 943–948.

Luria, A.R. (1966) *Higher Cortical Function in Man.* New York: Basic.

Maclean, P. (1992) 'The limbic system concept.' *In:* Trimble, M.R., Bolwig, T.G. (Eds.) *Temporal Lobes and Limbic System.* Petersfield: Wrightson Biomedical, pp. 1–14.

McGuire, P.K., Paulson, E., Frackowiak, R.S., Frith, C.D. (1996) *Neuroreport,* **7,** 2095–2099.

Nishizawa, Y., Olsen, T.S., Larsen, B., Lassen, N.A. (1982) 'Left–right cortical asymmetries of regional cerebral blood flow during listening to words.' *Journal of Neurophysiology,* **48,** 458–466.

O'Regan, M.E., Brown, J.K., Goodwin, G.M., Clarke, M. (1998) 'Epileptic aphasia: a consequence of regional hypometabolic encephalopathy.' *Developmental Medicine and Child Neurology,* **40,** 508–517.

O'Tuama, L.A., Urion, D.K., Janiek, M.J. (1992) 'Regional cerebral perfusion in Landau–Kleffner and related childhood aphasia.' *Journal of Nuclear Medicine,* **33,** 1758–1765.

Papez, J.W. (1937) 'A proposed mechanism of emotion.' *Archives of Neurology and Psychiatry,* **38,** 725–743.

Paul, R., Elwood, T.J. (1991) 'Maternal linguistic input to toddler with slow expressive language development.' *Journal of Speech and Hearing Research,* **34,** 982–988.

Penfield, W., Rasmussen, T. (1952) *The Cerebral Cortex of Man.* New York: Macmillan.

—— Roberts, L. (1959) *Speech and Brain Mechanisms.* Princeton: Princeton University Press.

Preis, S., Jancke, L., Schmitz-Hillebrecht, J., Steinmetz, H. (1999) 'Child age and planum temporale asymmetry.' *Brain and Cognition,* **40,** 441–452.

Price, C.J., Wise, R.J.S., Watson, J.D.G. (1994) 'Brain activity during reading: the effects of exposure, duration and task.' *Brain,* **117,** 1255–1269.

Rach, G.H., Zielhuis, G.A., Van der Brock, P. (1988) 'The influence of chronic persistent otitis media with effusion on language development of 2–4 year olds.' *International Journal of Pediatric Otorhinology,* **15,** 253–261.

Rossi, P.G., Parmoggiani, A., Posat, A., Scaduto, M.C., Chiodo, S., Vatti, G. (1999) 'Landau–Kleffner syndrome: long term follow up and links with electrical status in sleep (ESES).' *Brain and Development,* **21,** 90–98.

Rutter, M. (1980) 'The long term effect of early experience.' *Developmental Medicine and Child Neurology*, **22**, 800–815.

Smith, A. (1972) 'Dominant and non-dominant hemispherectomy.' *In:* Smith, W.L. (Ed.) *Drugs, Development and Cerebral Function.* Springfield, IL: C.C. Thomas, pp. 40–53.

Steinschneider, M., Volkov, I.O., Noh, M.D., Garell, P.C., Howard, M.A. (1999) 'Temporal encoding of the voice onset time phonetic parameter by field potentials recorded directly from human auditory cortex.' *Journal of Neurophysiology*, **82**, 2346—2357.

Strauss, E., Kosakon, B., Wada, J. (1983) 'The neurological basis of lateralised cerebral function.' *Human Neurobiology*, **2**, 115–127.

Wechsler, D. (1945) 'A standardized memory scale for clinical use.' *Journal of Psychology*, **19**, 87–95.

Zielhuis, G.A., Rach, G.A., van den Broek, P. (1989) 'Screening for otitis media with effusion in preschool children.' *Lancet*, **1**, 311–314.

2

THE NEUROLOGY OF SPEECH AND LANGUAGE DISORDERS IN CHILDREN. PART II: DISORDERS OF SPEECH

Mary E. O'Regan and J. Keith Brown

The average fully mature adult will have a vocabulary of some 10,000 words, an educated person 60,000 and one with a highly technical education 100,000, speaking at a rate of 165 words or 250 syllables per minute. A fast speaker may speak up to 300 words per minute. We can speak in English using only about 46 individual sounds (phonemes) and can represent the entire English language with combinations of 26 letters (graphemes). The development of speech in the young child has been studied extensively (Templin 1957, McNeill 1970, Ingram 1972, Rapin 1996), and we now have standardized tests of language comprehension, expression and pronunciation.

Section 2.1—Syntactical development

We have discussed in the previous chapter how we hear, understand and reason as a function of inner language. We speak to ourselves in our heads and hear this in the auditory association area of the superior temporal lobe; as we 'say to ourselves' this can now be seen on functional MRI. We activate the auditory association area in the temporal lobe whether the source of inner language that we are currently thinking about in consciousness arises from peripheral hearing, reading, sign language or abstract reasoning generated within our minds. We then have to decide on our response and equally 'inwardly hear' this before executing it as a motor action. We activate Broca's motor speech area when we say to ourselves during silent reading. There must therefore be a constant two-way communication, via the arcuate fasciculus, between the syntax in Broca's area and the 'inner hearing' of the planned reply in Wernicke's area. The grammatical construction of the sentence and its syntax are planned in Broca's area before being executed by sending instructions to the diaphragm, lips, tongue, palate and larynx on how to produce and sequence the relevant phonemes. Ultimately articulation is the physical medium through which spoken sentences are communicated.

BROCA'S AREA

The lips, tongue and palate are controlled via the corticobulbar tracts from the inferior end of the motor strip in the precentral gyrus (Fig. 2.1). The association area at the side of this primary motor area in the third frontal convolution is what is normally taken as Broca's area but it does extend into the insula. Although speech, which is learned, is usually localized

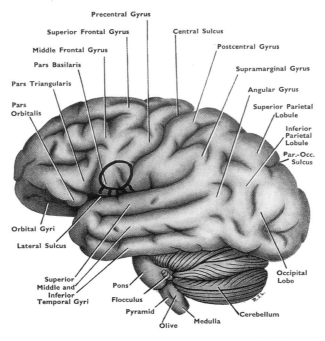

Fig. 2.1. Lateral surface of left hemisphere: note how Broca's area at the inferior end of the motor strip is part of the upper lip, *i.e.* operculum, of the lateral 'sylvian fissure' and extends inwards into the insula. (Adapted by permission from Last 1956.)

to Broca's area on the left, other functions of lips, tongue and palate such as bite, chew and swallow, which are innate, can be maintained by either side. However, a bilateral lesion, as with opercular dysplasia or herpes simplex late syndrome, causes not only loss of speech but also loss of bite, chew and swallow due to loss of both corticobulbar tracts.

The cerebral cortex is made up of modules that are, in reality, millions of individual learning units (Brown and Minns 1999). They have unique specificity of function even within what has often been taken to be an already specialized area of cortex, such as Broca's area. There are individual modules for nouns, verbs, and small words such as *it*, *at* and *so*. This means one can lose a particular part of language such as 'little word aphasia', a nominal aphasia for names, or only being able to speak in the present tense. Using PET with ^{15}O-labelled water as tracer, Wise *et al.* (1999) measured cerebral activity in 12 normal people performing three different tasks: repetition of heard nouns at different rates; listening to single nouns at different rates; and anticipation of listening or repetition. Repetition of single words did not activate Broca's area but activity was seen in three left lateralized regions: the anterior insula, a localized region in the lateral premotor cortex, and the posterior pallidum. The left anterior insula and lateral premotor cortex showed a conjunction of activity for hearing and articulation. Wise *et al.* concluded that the formulation of an articulatory

34

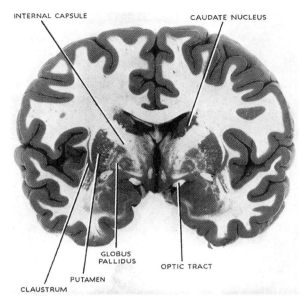

Fig. 2.2. Coronal section of brain at the level of the mammilary bodies. Note the amount of grey matter on the superior surface of the temporal lobe, *i.e.* Heschl's gyrus, and the amount of cortex in the insula forming part of Broca's area which cannot normally be seen from the outside of the brain. (Reproduced by permission from Last 1956.)

plan is a function of the left anterior insula and lateral premotor cortex and not of Broca's area alone. Using PET studies, Petersen *et al.* (1988) found that verb generation in response to a given noun increased perfusion in Broca's area. Linking nouns and verbs is at the heart of sentence production and involves mechanisms that lie well beyond the articulatory level. Mohr *et al.* (1978) studied 22 cases of stroke that clinically had a Broca's aphasia, using CT, angiography and autopsy records. They concluded that infarction of Broca's area alone does not produce a Broca's aphasia. To produce the clinical entity of Broca's aphasia a much larger lesion is required that encompasses the operculum including Broca's area, insula and adjacent cerebral cortex (Fig. 2.2). If one looks at the drawings of Broca's original specimens this is indeed the case, and the motor speech area is more extensive than the area adjacent to bulbar muscles in the motor strip.

Lateralization of Broca's area
Ninety per cent of the population are right-handed, and in most cases speech representation will be on the left side of the brain, although this is not invariable. Unilateral electroconvulsive therapy has shown that in over 90 per cent of right-handers speech is in the left hemisphere; in the remainder it is on the right side. One may therefore lose speech in association with a left hemiplegia. More rarely, Broca's area and Wernicke's area may be on opposite sides to each other—Broca's on the right and Wernicke's in its usual place on the left. Moreover,

there are many ambidextrous people, making strict division into right or left impossible; for instance, among 'left-handers' 60 per cent are definitely left-handed, about 20 per cent are ambidextrous, and 20 per cent use their left hand in order to write but use their right hand for most other tasks.

Of the 9 per cent of the population who are left-handed, around 60 per cent still have their speech on the left side of the brain. On Wada testing, seven out of 44 left-handed people were found to have bilateral representation of speech (Wada and Rasmussen 1960). In a study of regional cerebral blood flow during Wada testing, McMackin *et al.* (1998) found that among 13 patients with epilepsy, speech processing occurred in the left hemisphere in nine and in the right hemisphere in two, while in the remaining two it was bilateral. Injection of barbiturate into the left carotid artery caused greater hypoperfusion than when injected on the right. Most left-handed children have no specific learning disorder but there does seem to be a preponderance of left-handedness in reports of children with specific learning disorders. As Bishop (1980) points out, most males are not colour blind, but most colour-blind people are males, and equally it could be that the 7 per cent of left-handed people who have no definite localization of speech are more likely to have specific learning difficulties.

Boys are more strongly left-handed than are girls of a corresponding age, and this agrees with recent blood flow studies suggesting that language skills are more firmly unilateral in the male than in the female. Spatial skills are also thought to be established on average six years earlier in the male than in the female (Witelson 1976). One of the most dramatic new findings of functional MRI, which may contribute to the predominance of males among children with speech, language, reading and spelling problems, is that speech is very definitely localized to the left Broca's area in the male, while the female can use both hemispheres with bilateral representation (Reid *et al.* 1996).

Both sides of the brain can process speech and language, but there is normally a genetic bias to the left side of the brain and for right-handedness. If this gene is absent, then there is a random choice of handedness and a random chance for the placement of speech, so that 50 per cent may be right-handed and 50 per cent left-handed: this explains why a few people who are right-handed could process speech on the right side of their brain, why among monozygotic twins one may be right-handed and one left-handed, and why 70 per cent of children are right-handed even when both parents are left-handed.

NORMAL SYNTACTICAL DEVELOPMENT

Children's understanding precedes their ability to speak, and very young infants can be taught a manual signing system before they can articulate. Simple naming of objects is the first language ability to manifest in the second year of life and necessitates the mental association of a visual object with a heard name. The child in the third year then learns characteristics of these objects such as number, colour, size (big or small), shape (square, triangle, etc.), position (in, out, beside), taste (nice or nasty) and smell. Nowadays this is strongly reinforced by television programmes, videos, simple computer games, books and comics. The child also learns to recognize identity such as boy or girl, *I* am *me* (also *I* do things, *i.e.* one uses *I* not *me* before a verb), *you* are *mummy*, and so forth. S/he thus learns the characteristics of common objects, *i.e.* is developing concepts; understanding auditory/visual associations is essential, and any visual or auditory perception problem will prevent this. The right cerebral hemisphere will perceive the object and this must be connected across the splenium of the corpus callosum to the language area on the opposite side. Corpus callosotomy will prevent this and so a person could not then associate the sound of a film with the pictures.

Grammar has to be learned. At first the child will learn simple rules that s/he will apply in all situations, *e.g.* in plurals one adds an *-s* at the end of the word (*foots, sheeps, mouses*), and the past tense is indicated by adding *-ed* (*comed, goed, wented*). There is also difficulty with time—*today, tomorrow, yesterday*—and with pronouns such as *I* for *me*.

Syntax develops from single words meaning a whole utterance (holophrastic speech, *e.g. ta-ta, mum, poo, moo-moo*) to a strictly structured two-word system known as 'open' or 'pivot' words: the open words could be *mummy, moon, dog, juice, place*, and the pivot words, *all gone, big, more, pretty, bye-bye*, so that we would get "all gone mummy", "all gone moon", "all gone juice", "all gone dog", etc. This two-word system is then gradually replaced by simple phrase structure. At 2.5 years of age the child uses an average of three and a maximum of eight words per utterance, and 95 per cent of these words are in the simple present tense. By 3 years s/he uses an average of six words per utterance and 15 in the longest sentence, and there are now three times more verbs in the past tense (McNeil 1970).

By the end of the second year the child can understand simple *what, where, when* type questions. By the end of the third year s/he understands concepts such as prepositions, quantity, colour and size of objects. During the second year vocabulary is small and 'over-extensions' occur, *e.g.* all animals are called "cat". In the third year vocabulary increases rapidly to an average of 1000 words (O'Hare and Brown 1997).

Between 3 and 5 years comprehension becomes increasingly complex, *e.g.* adjectives and descriptive words are recognized (*wet/dry, hot/cold, large/small, beside/inside*) and the function of objects is also understood. At school entry, normal children can understand three-part instructions, are less dependent on context and are developing abstract understanding, *e.g.* time.

EXPRESSIVE DYSPHASIA

A developmental syntactical dysphasia, *i.e.* slow development of grammatical sentence construction, is usually accompanied by a delay in phonological development, *i.e.* word pronunciation, as part of the genetic developmental speech disorder syndrome. Occasionally one sees pure syntactical dysphasias, usually of genetic origin. Comprehension must be normal and well advanced on the level of speech development or the probability is of mild learning disability, deafness or word deafness. The clinical picture consists of a slowing up of the normal development described above, *i.e.* single words persist for a long time with short telegrammatic sentences, the mean length of utterance is reduced, pronoun reversal occurs (*e.g. me* for *I*), and past tenses and plurals cause difficulty. On sentence repetition, even well on in school age, words are omitted and parts of the sentence are reversed. Time concepts such as *yesterday, today, tomorrow* or *in a minute* are difficult to grasp.

ACQUIRED EXPRESSIVE DYSPHASIA

The concept of an aphasia produced by infarction of Broca's area has become so entrenched

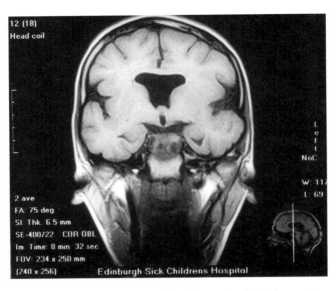

Fig. 2.3. Developmental abnormality of a child's brain with opercular dysplasia exposing an area of speech cortex normally hidden: dysplasia causes a Worster Drought type of mixed cortical bulbar palsy with aphasia.

in classical neurology that it is now a fundamental dictum. An expressive aphasia in children is most commonly due to trauma from road traffic accidents in which the sphenoid wing causes local laceration and contusion; more rarely it occurs from cerebrovascular disease or tumours. A specific encephalitis of the opercular region of the insula and superior temporal gyrus occurs with reactivation of a previous herpes encephalitis, and similar damage has been suggested from status epilepticus. As road traffic accidents decrease, epileptic aphasias become increasingly important. In 25 such children studied by O'Regan *et al.* (1998) a mixed picture was found: 20 had an expressive dysphasia, eight had nominal difficulties, and 10 had articulatory dyspraxia.

The lesion is usually at the lower end of the motor strip, in the operculum and extending into the insula. A bilateral perisylvian (*i.e.* opercular) dysplasia is seen in some children (Worster Drought syndrome, see below) who show bilateral facial palsy, palatal palsy and severe expressive speech difficulty (Fig. 2.3). This is easily confused with Moebius syndrome, from a brainstem dysplasia, when a VIth nerve weakness always accompanies the bilateral facial weakness. In adults with expressive aphasia, a poor prognosis for recovery is related to damage to deep white matter at the lateral angle of the frontal horn (deep in Broca's area and affecting projections from the cingulate gyrus and the premotor strip to the caudate nucleus). This may have some relevance in children, in whom damage to periventricular white matter is relatively common (Naeser *et al.* 1989).

There are similarities in the speech of children and of adults with Broca's aphasia, but in severe cases there is inability to utter or write a single word. Initial mutism is followed by word finding difficulties, with disorganization of syntax structure in speech, writing and pronunciation; this affects spontaneous speech, sentence repetition and reading aloud. Affected persons know the correct word when it is chosen from a group of words or even when lip-read from the examiner; they cannot read aloud but may be able to read silently to themselves.

Speech is similar to that of a 2-year-old, consisting of single nouns or verbs, *i.e.* holophrastic speech, without adjectives, adverbs or articles. Verbs tend to be in one tense, like *gone*, *come*, *go*, and nouns are usually in the singular. Counting, reciting the days of the week, and automatic speech ("Oh my!" "Oh dear!" "Damn it!") as well as emotional speech, such as swearing, may be preserved. Some patients lose very specific parts of speech such as with the so-called 'little word aphasia' where words like *on*, *in*, *at* and *it* may be lost, though *yes* and *no* can be preserved in isolation. Specific groups of words may be lost, *e.g.* words describing position (*inside*, *beside*, *up/down*). Sentences are shortened and words left out, *i.e.* telegrammatic speech. Paraphrasias may occur with substitutions of well-articulated phonemes or words (verbal paraphrasias). If substitutions become numerous following the mutism, jargon aphasia may result with words becoming unrecognizable or the invention of new words that do not occur in the language (neologisms) (Van Hout *et al.* 1985).

Section 2.2—Phonological development: motor learning of speech

Each part of the human body is represented by the homunculus lying along the precentral motor strip, with the lips, tongue and palate having a large representation (Fig. 2.4). It is not known whether the large part of the motor strip that is given over to the mouth and hands developed so that speech and hand manipulation were then possible, or whether very frequent use of part of the body causes overgrowth of the corresponding part of the brain. In the pig the whole motor strip is taken up by the snout. In violinists, it has been shown that the finger area of the fingering hand is overdeveloped (Elbert *et al.* 1995), and Einstein's brain had overdevelopment of the parietal area (Galaburda 1999), suggesting that constant use does cause focal hypertrophy. The fact that in congenital hemiplegia the loss of part of the motor strip on the opposite side to the weak hand can be compensated for by development of a new motor area on the same side as the weakness suggests there is enough plasticity to change brain morphology by practice.

Each part of the body has an association area adjacent to it. This area is responsible for storing the memories of learned skills, *i.e.* an engram of movement sequences, so-called 'kinaesthetic memory'. This area 6 of Brodman has strong connections with the cerebellum, basal ganglia and reticular formation. Loss of ability in area 6 lesions impairs motor learning for the particular strategy, *i.e.* causes an apraxia such as articulatory dyspraxia, constructional dyspraxia or writing dyspraxia. Damage to these areas may produce the tendency to continue a certain movement even though the movement is unsuccessful in achieving its goal (perseveration).

CEREBELLAR FUNCTION

The cerebellum receives a vast amount of sensory information from the muscle spindles,

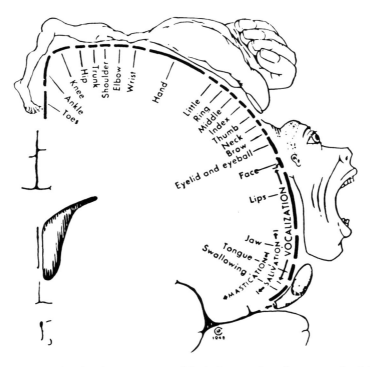

Fig. 2.4. Homunculus showing the arrangement of the body parts along the motor strip of the cerebral cortex.

tendon organs, labyrinths, eyes and skin proprioceptors, as well as the cortex itself, and yet there is no sensory loss in cerebellar disease. It possesses 40 times more input than output fibres and contains 50 per cent of all neurons. It is thought that certain sensory information such as that from the muscle spindles is only indirectly available to the motor cortex through the cerebellum, and in turn a very large part of the output from the motor cortex is to the cerebellum.

It is thought that there is point-to-point somatotrophic representation between cerebral cortex and cerebellar cortex. Information about a movement of, say, lips, tongue and palate being planned by the cerebral cortex passes to the Purkinje cells of the cerebellum. These have a vast arborization of dendrites in contact with all the incoming sensory information outlined above. This is computed and the information then sent back to the cerebral cortex. It has a function to make the decision on what force, speed, direction and distance are required by the muscles to most smoothly execute the movement planned by the cortex. It is thought also to be important in motor learning, especially of automatic motor tasks, and therefore in learning the motor engrams necessary for speech. *i.e.* muscle movements for the production of phonemes. This can lead to slow speech development and an ataxic dysarthria in children with cerebellar damage.

There is also a syndrome of cerebellar 'mutism' that occurs in children following re-section of cerebellar tumours, probably due to the disruption of motor learning necessary for phoneme production: the mutism is followed by a dysarthria that is slow and hypernasal. It is most common after surgery for midline vermis tumours such as primitive neuroectodermal tumours (Catsman-Berrevoets *et al.* 1999). Catsman-Berrevoets and Van Dongen (1997) studied 42 children with cerebellar tumours using structural and functional imaging pre- and post-operatively: 12 developed postoperative mutism, and SPECT revealed frontal hypoperfusion bilaterally in these patients. Further SPECT studies (Germano *et al.* 1998) in two children who developed transient mutism following posterior fossa tumour resection showed a marked reduction of cerebral perfusion in the right fronto-parietal region in one child and a reduction in perfusion in the left fronto-parietal region in the other. When these children regained normal speech, follow-up SPECT revealed normalization of the cerebral perfusion.

BASAL GANGLIA FUNCTION

The basal ganglia, like the cerebellum, have a loop system with the cerebral cortex. The basal ganglia are regarded as extrapyramidal as they affect muscles through a different pathway than the corticospinal, *i.e.* the pyramidal pathway. In this way, two messages can be sent simultaneously to a group of muscles. The expression of emotion in the right hemisphere can therefore be superimposed upon the logical thoughts of language from the left, *e.g.* intonation is imposed upon speech, expression on piano playing and emotional rhythm onto dance steps. Just as the cerebellum sends messages back to the cerebral cortex for regulation of the force, speed, distance, etc. of the movement being planned, so the basal ganglia control smooth flow, speed (cadence), start, stop, pauses, stress and emotional overtones of the movement being planned. The output is therefore mainly back to the cerebral cortex and only in abnormal circumstances directly to the spinal cord.

The cadence of motor actions such as the speed of speech, speed of writing and elective walking speed are determined by this system. Lesions of the basal ganglia produce delay in initiating speech, with slow, laboured production lacking smooth flow and the normal imperceptible blending of pauses and stress, lack of prosody causing monotonous speech with little variation in pitch. The clinical features of an extrapyramidal bulbar palsy are described below in the section on dysarthrias (pp. 59–60).

Stammering is a speech dysrhythmia that affects fluency, start/stop and flow as well as changing cadence, suggesting a basal ganglia type of disorder. The child most commonly has difficulty in starting a new word or phrase and will either block (so that no sound comes out), prolong the first syllable, or repeat the first syllable or whole word (stammer). Repetitions tend to develop before the blocks and prolongations. Most affected individuals come to recognize particular words in a sentence that will cause them difficulty. Long words giving meaning at the beginning of a sentence are most likely to cause problems, but there is no particular group of words in the English language that is common to all stammerers as likely to cause particular difficulty. Establishing a rhythm will help many extrapyramidal disorders, not just stammering.

The speed of speaking varies with the individual, and either from excitement or in order to stress certain words or emphasize a piece of information, the speed may increase.

Speech is slow in basal ganglia diseases such as parkinsonism. While slow speech may be used deliberately to create a feeling of importance or gravity, a rate of speech of less than 60 words per minute (wpm) sounds very slow and becomes difficult to hold in short-term memory in order to extract meaning. Speeds over 300 wpm (as may happen in the case of racing commentators) cause difficulty in sustaining attention and the speech may become incomprehensible. Very rapid speech may occur in some very young children when they 'fall over themselves' in speech, so-called 'cluttering'.

Section 2.3—Speech production

Speech requires: (1) an airflow; (2) voice; (3) palatal shunting of airflow; and (4) precise tongue and lip movements (articulation).

AIRFLOW

Airflow is supplied by the diaphragm producing a steady flow of air during expiration. Without this there would be a tremulant effect and variation in volume. The natural tendency to regular automatic breathing must be suspended as airflow is obstructed in certain consonants (*p*, *b*, *g*), but must also stop and start to allow the pauses in speech and to signal start and stop of words. There is a higher centre for respiratory control in the frontal lobe (middle frontal gyrus) adjacent to Broca's area and the insula that allows coordination of breathing and speech. Breathlessness in heart disease, chronic lung disease or severe anxiety produces short sentences with deep inspiration.

VOICE

The larynx has two functions: firstly a sphincter action to protect the respiratory tract from aspiration of food, and secondly, phonation. Phonation can occur without a larynx (as is seen in oesophageal speech). Sound is produced by a vibrating air stream because of the vibrations set up in the vocal cords. The cords themselves do not produce speech, merely a noise, which without resonation of the nasal cavities (rhinophony), pharynx and chest would sound quite thin and reedy. The air stream pressure causes the cords to vibrate only when they are proximate and when they are contracted; it is not a free vibration of loose cords in the air stream. The tension in the cords will vary the pitch; changing breath stream pressure will alter the volume.

The cricothyroid muscle is the main muscle that causes lengthening of the vocal cord, while the thyroarytenoid (which includes the vocalis muscle) shortens the cords. All the intrinsic muscles of the larynx are supplied from the medulla, having their origin in the nucleus ambiguus. The cricothyroid muscle takes its innervation from the superior laryngeal nerve, which is a branch of the vagus nerve in the neck, and sometimes has some fibres from the spinal accessory nerve, while all the other muscles of the larynx are supplied by the recurrent laryngeal nerve which branches from the vagus, looping on the right side of the body around the right subclavian artery, while on the left it loops at the level of the left ligamentum arteriosum. Both nerves in the neck lie in the groove between the trachea and the oesophagus and so are vulnerable during thyroid surgery. In cases of recurrent laryngeal nerve palsy, the abductor muscles of the larynx are affected first (Semon's law), so that the vocal cord on the affected side moves toward the midline. As the recurrent laryngeal nerve palsy becomes complete, the cord comes to lie in the so-called cadaveric abducted position. If the lesion is unilateral, the opposite cord gradually manages to oppose the paralysed cord so that the hoarseness will diminish, but if the paresis is bilateral, persistent aphonia will result.

The voice shows obvious pitch differences between male and female particularly after puberty, and normal speech shows wide swings of pitch so we sing as we speak (see above). The volume of a voice varies in normal speech in order to stress a point; phonation helps to indicate nationality or dialect. The voice is also repeatedly switched on and off, independent of breathing, so that all vowels are voiced, as well as some consonants (*m, n, l, j, z*), while others have the voice switched off (*s, t, th, sh, k*).

Dysphonia

Dysphonia presents as a gruff, deep voice with loss of ability to sing high tones or no voice with the patient only able to articulate in a whisper. Diagnosis has been aided by the use of fibre-optic laryngoscopes and MRI. Dysphonia can result from an anatomical abnormality of the larynx, from a neurological lesion affecting its innervation or the muscles themselves, or from psychological factors.

The cords may be involved in malignant tumours such as the embryonal variant of rhabdomyosarcoma of the larynx, or benign polyps and cysts. Radiation *in utero* or for benign laryngeal nodules can predispose to malignant laryngeal tumours (Ferlito *et al.* 1999). The vocal cords may be thickened and have nodules as a result of excessive/incorrect use of the voice (so-called 'singer's nodules'), which in children are more likely to be due to constant screaming and shouting, or effortful phonation as may be seen in cerebral palsy. Acute laryngitis results in hoarseness, breathiness, loss of high tones, a drop in pitch, loss of pitch swings, eventual aphonia and, in severe cases, stridor. The two commonest reasons nowadays for chronic laryngeal inflammation causing dysphonia are probably: (i) a chemical irritation from hydrochloric acid, due to gastro-oesophageal reflux—this is not uncommon if 24 hour pH studies are performed in children with dysphonia (Bouchard *et al.* 1999); and (ii) the use of inhaled steroids in asthma, since the use of a spacer increases lung and decreases pharyngeal deposition (Jackson *et al.* 1999). Thrush of the pharynx and larynx often complicates these latter cases. Chronic involvement of the cords occurs in tuberculosis; they may be thickened in myxoedema when the voice is deep and sounds as though the patient is talking through a mouthful of food. Tumours such as haemangiomas of the subglottic region may splint the vocal cords, preventing free movement and causing dysphonia. Trauma to the larynx can occur from accidental hanging, from prolonged intratracheal intubation as in the preterm neonate resulting in subglottic stenosis, or from drinking caustics.

The larynx may be congenitally abnormal with a glottic web or in some of the craniofacial syndromes such as Goldenhar syndrome and occasionally Treacher–Collins syndrome. There is a rare familial type of dysphonia, inherited as an autosomal recessive condition, in which there may be no phonation and the child communicates by whispering. Dysphonia with a harsh, gruff, low-frequency voice is a common manifestation in children with Down syndrome.

Neurological dysphonia
The laryngeal muscles will weaken with prolonged use of the voice in myasthenia gravis. The recurrent laryngeal nerve may be injured during neck surgery (especially thyroid surgery or removal of a cystic hygroma) or chest surgery, being especially vulnerable on the left side where it runs round the aortic arch. It can be trapped in suppurating hilar lymph nodes. The vagus nerve is more likely to be involved in compression by tumours of the nasopharynx spreading into the base of the skull through the jugular foramen—this could result in complete paralysis of the pharynx with associated dysarthria and dysphagia. Both vagal nuclei can be affected in brainstem infarction and secondary brainstem haemorrhage as in children with head injuries or pontine gliomas. Aphonia may rarely arise as an hysterical symptom, especially in teenagers.

PALATAL FUNCTION
The soft palate can shunt the airflow so that it all enters the nasopharynx and none comes out of the mouth, adding resonance to the voice that would otherwise be thin and reedy. There should be no nasal escape if the child says "e-e-e-e", all airflow being by the mouth—*i.e.* if one pinches the nose while the child phonates there should be no modulation of the sound. When s/he says "n-n-n-n" all airflow should be through the nose. In palatal palsies, in short palate following cleft palate repairs, and in submucous clefts, there is hyperrhino-phonia (hypernasal speech) and the palate cannot close off the nasopharynx so air escapes. The palate is paralysed in diphtheria and in brainstem tumours such as pontine gliomas, and a rare type of parainfectious polyneuritis may cause palatal palsy. In adenoidal hyper-trophy, hyporhinophonia occurs with the opposite effect. Palatal movements while saying "n-n-n-n" and "e-e-e-e" can be shown by X-ray palatography or viewed by a pernasal endoscope. The nasopharynx can now be seen in detail by MRI, and real time MRI during speech is likely to completely replace other methods in the future (Fig. 2.5).

ARTICULATION
Articulation by the lips, tongue and palate requires an ability to make precise movements rapidly and in sequence. For instance, consider the sequence of movements of the tongue required when saying a simple word like "loss". The tongue, which appears anatomically as a single big bunch of muscle, has to be controlled very accurately: the tongue tip is opposed to the palate in "l"; the tongue is then flattened to the floor of the mouth for "o"; and then a precise area behind the tip must be reapplied to the palate for "ss". This requires the same amount of skill and coordination as in very fine hand skills. Figure 2.6, of a series of plasticine models designed in the late 19th century by Lord Rayleigh to demonstrate the movements of the mouth during speech (known as 'Lord Rayleigh's organ'), illustrates how physicians of the time were intrigued by the alterations in the shape of the mouth necessary for articulation (Paget 1930, Ghazala 1993).

KINAESTHETIC MEMORY: THE MOTOR ENGRAM
The learning of how to say a simple word such as "spoon" requires a learned motor sequence, *i.e.* an engram to be stored in motor (kinaesthetic) memory. This would entail a sophisticated

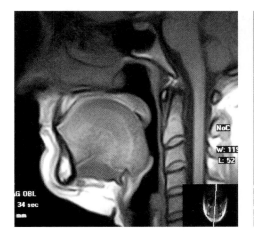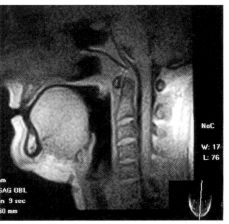

Fig. 2.5. MRI palatograms showing (a) the occlusion of the buccal airway by bunching the tongue against the hard palate and lowering the soft palate thus opening the nasopharynx when saying "n-n-n-n", and (b) closing the nasal airway by elevating the soft palate and opening the buccal airway when saying "e-e-e-e". (New high-definition scanners give even better definition.)

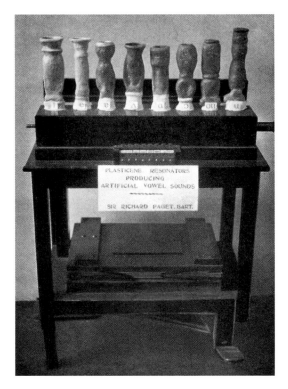

Fig. 2.6. Lord Rayleigh's organ of plasticine models showing the various shapes of the mouth and pharynx necessary to articulate the vowels. (Reproduced from Paget 1930.)

set of instructions to voice, diaphragm, lips, tongue and palate. The diagram below shows the sequence of signals from the motor strip to the muscles of lips, tongue, palate, breathing and voice needed to say the word "spoon": the tune to be played by Broca on the rolandic piano (the central sulcus is the fissure of Rolando). A different series of signals will be required to the small muscles of the hand and wrist from the graphomotor area in order to write the word spoon. This grouping of motor memories for a sequence of movements into an engram is exactly the same as the grouping of cognitive memories into a concept but utilizes completely different brain circuits, requires repetition and practice, and is not dependent upon a language.

	Lips	Tongue	Palate	Voice	Breath
S	−	+	−	−	+
P	+	+	−	−	−
O	+	−	−	+	+
O	+	−	−	+	+
N	−	+	+	+	+

Development of the primary motor area of the cortex, corticobulbar tract, association area of Broca, supplementary motor area, cerebellum and basal ganglia are all essential for the learning of these sequenced motor skills. The rate at which development proceeds is influenced by the sex of the child, genetic factors and brain damage. With practice, the speed of a motor act increases; with further practice, it becomes automatic, and so subconscious, at which time emotional overtones can be added.

NORMAL SPEECH DEVELOPMENT
By the time children produce their first word with meaning (50th centile 12 months, 90th centile 18 months) they have already developed complex preverbal communication and can produce all the individual sounds required for speech. During their first six months, infants learn to distinguish between speech and non-speech sounds and can differentiate intonation (auditory discrimination). They can produce consonant/vowel single-syllable babble: *ma-ma-ma*, *ga-ga-ga*. During the second six months they start to recognize their name and those of other family members, and babbling becomes increasingly complex. By the end of the first year they use many consistent sound sequences to represent 'protowords', and these, combined with increasing use of nonverbal features such as eye pointing and gesture, increase their ability to communicate.

Between 12 and 18 months, children can sequence only a limited range of consonants—*b, d, m, n, p, t*—with vowels as in *mama, papa, dada, nana, ta-ta, bye-bye, pee-pee, poo, moo-moo, baba*, etc. This gradually increases in sophistication with acquisition of an increasing number of consonants so that by 2 to 3 years they can sequence a wider range including *f, g, h, j, k, l, s* and *w*, which at first they are able to put only into certain parts of a word and before or after certain consonants or blends. In other situations they will omit the sound or substitute one that they can make (*d/g, d/j, l/r, s/i, t/k, t/th*) for the so-called later-acquired consonant (*ch, dge, f, g, k, l, r, sh, th*).

Phonological development normally proceeds in a predictable manner. Most of the later-acquired speech sounds, at least in connective speech, are fricative sounds like *s* and *f*, or sounds that can be prolonged such as *r* and *l*. There is therefore a pattern to speech that is consistent if one understands the omissions, insertions, reversals and substitutions being used, which is known as a developmental pattern. The paediatrician can recognize characteristic developmental patterns of omissions (*poon/spoon*), substitutions (*lolly/lorry*, *yeyow/yellow*), reversals (*aminals/animals*, *ephelan/elephant*) and insertions (*plegs/pegs*).

The mirror image learning in both hemispheres means that reversals of sounds in words and reversals of words in phrases are added to the immature motor performance. Other young children will often be able to understand the child with developmental speech problems better than adults can, and a sibling may translate so that the parents feel that their child is just lazy, having no need to speak. In most cases this is untrue. A child may say, for instance, "poon" for "spoon" and yet be able to make the sound *s* in isolation. This is the way that a child acquires the motor skill and is not laziness. The child will often point or gesture and make a lot of facial grimacing. Between 3 and 4 years, phonology matures but some normal children continue to show difficulties with consonant clusters, especially if they can be prolonged such as *ch* or *sh*. By the age of 5 the phonological development is largely complete, and although there may still be problems with *r*, *l* and *th*, the speech is entirely intelligible (O'Hare and Brown 1997).

DELAYED SPEECH DEVELOPMENT
The reported incidence in the population of a significant slowing down of speech development, as described above, depends on the criteria used. If all children are included, then 1.8 per cent of boys and 0.9 per cent of girls will remain unintelligible at the age of 7 years, with a preponderance from socially disadvantaged and large families (Butler *et al.* 1973). However, 50 per cent of children who are language delayed at 30 months will be retarded in nonverbal abilities on follow-up (Silva 1980). The incidence of severe specific speech and language disorder, defined as only a few single words at 3 years and limited connected speech at 5 years, but average intelligence, is one per 1000 (Ingram 1973). Stevenson and Richman (1976) found an overall incidence of slow speech at 3 years of 3 per cent and severe disorder in between two and five per 1000. Against all these figures it must be remembered that speech development follows a normal distribution curve with 10 per cent of children falling below the 10th centile and 3 per cent below the third centile, and these children are not necessarily 'abnormal' in relation to their peers.

CAUSES OF DELAYED LEARNING OF SPEECH
All the causes of slowing down of normal brain development are illustrated by slowing of speech development. All children with generalized learning difficulty will be slow to speak. Ambidextrousness, left-earedness, signs of delayed dominance, environmental deprivation and genetic factors have all been stressed (Ingram 1959). Environmental factors are obviously of immense importance as the child can only learn the speech that s/he has heard. Deafness, particularly high-tone deafness, must be considered in every case. Glue ear with temporary deafness is incriminated as a cause of slowed speech development and this may be more obvious in phonology than in understanding (Abraham *et al.* 1996). Brain damage will also slow the rate of speech acquisition, so that about 25 per cent of preterm infants or of those

asphyxiated at birth will have slow speech development sufficient to require speech therapy. Many children with ataxia, *e.g.* following hydrocephalus or associated with hypothyroidism, have slowing of motor learning and thus of expressive speech development. Forty per cent of children with a congenital hemiplegia will have delay in maturation of speech and not a dysarthria or dysphasia. Robinson (1991) found in a study of 82 school-age children with slow speech development that genetic factors were predominant in 50 per cent; another 26 per cent had identifiable causes—11 per cent prenatal, 3 per cent perinatal and 12 per cent postnatal, including five with epileptic aphasia.

Males with the disorder outnumber females by 3:1; the whole of the left cerebral hemisphere is thought to mature more slowly in boys due to the effects of the Y chromosome. The frontal pole and the angular gyrus areas are called terminal or tertiary zones and are the last parts of the cerebral cortex to mature, after birth, and are more likely to be affected by any generalized brain insult such as hypoxia or trauma or by preterm birth. Hyperkinesis, attention deficit from frontal pole delay, and slow speech and reading from delayed development of the angular gyrus would therefore be expected to result. Radiation *in utero* can be shown to selectively affect the left cerebral hemisphere and hence speech and language development (Loganovskaja and Loganovsky 1999). Not only will the motor aspects of speech be retarded, but syntax and semantics will also be affected to some degree and in a few cases to a severe degree.

Disorders in children tend to be more generalized, such as preterm birth, asphyxia or chromosome disorders (XYY, XXO, fragile X), indicating that the rate of development of the whole brain is affected rather than one specific part. Children with Down syndrome will also show a developmental type of speech disorder (Van Borsel 1988). Developmental disorders of speech and language do not separate into strictly defined entities as readily as the acquired disorders do. Equally the development of specific modules in the cerebral cortex must be under genetic control and so can be affected in isolation by genetic disease; one does see children in whom the disorder is purely phonological (dyslalia or articulatory dyspraxia), predominantly syntactical, or involving semantics as described above under receptive dysphasia. In Scotland certain families relating to the old clan system are known to have a higher incidence of developmental speech retardation, and again, in Ingram's original studies, of 75 cases of speech retardation a parent was similarly affected in 18 cases and a sibling in 24 cases (Ingram 1959). Twin studies suggest genetic and not perinatal factors are most important (Bishop 1997). If parents are asked to repeat difficult-to-articulate phrases and sentences, difficulty is shown to persist into adult life. Lewis and Fairbairn (1998) looked at 38 school-age siblings and 94 parents of index children with phonological delay: although great improvements occurred over time, those parents with a definite history of slow speech still showed abnormality as adults. This type of examination would greatly enhance future genetic studies as the same authors found there was no outstanding clinical difference between the 58 per cent of speech-retarded children with a positive family history and the 42 per cent with no family history.

The speech of affected children shows the omissions, substitutions, reversals and insertions seen in normal speech development but over a much more elongated time scale. They have fewer correctly pronounced consonants, and the percentage of intelligible utterances is reduced, as is the mean length of utterance. Most children will have difficulty with the later acquired fricative sounds such as *th*, *rr* and *sh*, persisting into school years, but speech should be mature by 7 to 8 years—if not, problems are very likely to continue in the long term. In these latter cases later language function as tested by vocabulary and language comprehension is usually normal, although phonological processing and reading may still show persisting abnormalities at 15 to 16 years (Stothard *et al.* 1998). If the pattern is atypical (as demonstrated by the Edinburgh articulation test) then an articulatory dyspraxia with persisting difficulty is more likely. The prognosis therefore depends upon how rapidly acquisition of consonants occurs after 3 years of age, whether the pattern is typical, and whether it is specific, *i.e.* whether there are also abnormalities of nonverbal intelligence. Children having disorders of inner language, *i.e.* with specific language impairment, rather than a pure phonological problem, are very likely to show persisting problems in syntax, *e.g.* sentence repetition, reading and spelling (Ingram 1972, Burden *et al.* 1996). They show continued phonological problems when trying to phonetically analyse words, match phoneme to grapheme, or match words that begin with the same sound or words that rhyme—hence the relationship to dyslexia (Ingram 1972, Brown and Minns 1999).

Articulatory dyspraxia
When phonology is severely disturbed, the clinical picture merges into that of an articulatory dyspraxia (Ferry *et al.* 1975). Children with simple phonological delay may show dyspraxia or clumsiness in hand manipulation and postural control (Owen and McKinley 1997). Children with articulatory dyspraxia are distinguished by their poor prognosis for the development of speech. Lou *et al.* (1984) demonstrated decreased blood flow in the lower part of the premotor cortex (Broca's area) in three such children. PET activation study revealed functional abnormalities in both cortical and subcortical motor-related areas of the frontal lobe, while quantitative MRI analysis revealed structural abnormalities in several of these areas, particularly the caudate nucleus which was found to be abnormally small bilaterally.

There is increasing evidence that articulatory dyspraxia has a genetic basis. Vargha-Khadem *et al.* (1998) have described a three-generation family, half of whose members are affected by a pronounced verbal dyspraxia. A recent linkage study (Fisher *et al.* 1998) localized the abnormal gene (*SPCH1*) to a 5.6 centimorgan interval in the chromosome band 7q31. The genetic mutation or deletion in this region has resulted in the abnormal development of several brain areas that appear to be critical for both orofacial movements and sequential articulation. Scheffer *et al.* (1995) described a family of nine affected individuals in three generations with nocturnal partial seizures (benign rolandic epilepsy) affecting the face and arms with, in addition, oral and speech dyspraxia. The speech disorder was prominent but differed from that seen in Landau–Kleffner syndrome and ESES (see above). The EEG was also abnormal, showing features resembling autosomal dominant rolandic epilepsy. This family also showed clinical anticipation of the seizure disorder and of the oral and speech dyspraxia, suggesting that the genetic mechanism could be expansion of an unstable triplet repeat.

In a minority of cases, there may be some nasal escape in speech but the palate will move well with "ah" and the gag reflex is normal. However, the soft palate does not close off the nasopharynx during connected speech and this may cause misdiagnosis of mild

TABLE 2.1
Forms of dysarthria

Anatomical dysarthria
Neurological dysarthria
    Spastic dysarthria (pseudobulbar palsy)
    Flaccid dysarthria (true bulbar palsy and myopathies)
    Extrapyramidal or dyskinetic dysarthria
        Hypokinetic
        Hyperkinetic
    Ataxic dysarthria

pseudobulbar palsy. The pattern of speech is often deviant with bizarre omissions and substitutions that are inconsistent and may involve vowels as well as consonants. As the child matures s/he may be able to make most of the 46 speech sounds in isolation but cannot sequence them into words. Imitation of speech may be more accurate than spontaneous speech, suggesting an intact inner representation of phonology. There will be some words that s/he learns and articulates very well, *i.e.* s/he may overlearn a few words or phrases. When s/he is anxious speech will disintegrate further, and when speaking quickly it will become even less understandable. A specific speech sound may be used in one word and not in another. In very severe cases the child may not even be able to imitate certain individual sounds. S/he may learn to say a simple word such as "cat" and yet when trying to say "catapult" cannot even pronounce the "cat-" distinctly. In severe cases the child may circumvent the articulation problem by contracting sentences so that speech become telegrammatic, often consisting of one- or two-word utterances. Some children may also have oromotor dyspraxia, *e.g.* they cannot imitate rapid repetitive lateral movements of the tongue. In addition, girls in particular may have an upper limb dyspraxia that presents problems when learning a manual signing system to augment communication. However, there is not always a strict relationship between manual and articulatory dyspraxia (Kornse *et al.* 1981).

Acquired articulatory dyspraxia
In its fully developed form this is very similar to the congenital type. There is difficulty with speech sounds, especially consonant blends with inconsistent substitutions or omissions. Word synthesis is slow, problems occurring more with the beginning of words than the end. Long words cause particular difficulty; individual syllables may be pronounced in isolation but cannot be sequenced together, *e.g. wheel* and *barrow* but not *wheelbarrow*. The child's comprehension may be normal and there may not be any word-finding difficulty, unless there is an additional expressive dysphasia. S/he knows what s/he wants to say and knows that her/his pronunciation is abnormal. Acquired articulatory dyspraxia is usually caused by small lesions in the region of the inferior frontal gyrus of the dominant hemisphere due to vascular lesions, small tumours, bullet wounds, etc.

THE DYSARTHRIAS
The various types of dysarthria are listed in Table 2.1.

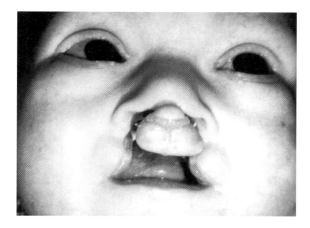

Fig. 2.7. Hare lip and cleft palate. The short palate after closure can cause a severe anatomical dysarthria with nasal escape and recurrent otitis media.

Anatomical causes of dysarthria

Abnormalities of the tongue are usually overemphasized as a cause of speech disorders, especially in folklore. Children with congenital abnormalities of the tongue may have hemiglossectomies and still have completely normal speech. It has even been suggested that people with congenital aglossia can have intelligible speech.

The commonest cause of dysarthria due to an anatomical lesion is cleft palate syndrome (Fig. 2.7). If the palate is not intact, the soft palate does not close off the nasal cavity completely, and intrabuccal pressure cannot then be increased to produce certain sounds such as *p*, *b* or *t*, or those requiring a sustained air flow such as *s* or *ee*. Instead, the air escapes through the nose, and may be heard during speech as nasal escape. Slow and difficult feeding, especially with regurgitation through the nose, should suggest the possibility of a cleft or submucous cleft palate. The palate itself may have a submucous cleft as indicated by a bifid uvula or can be congenitally short as part of the malformation. An inadequate repair or postoperative infection may have caused fibrosis and subsequent contraction. Acquired palatal disorders, such as injury from falling on a sharp object while holding it in the mouth, can result in contraction from scarring. If the palate does not close completely, the eustachian tubes may not be protected so that reflux or obstruction will predispose to chronic secretory otitis and conductive deafness that further aggravates the speech disorder. The palate may be congenitally short with or without a submucous cleft; removal of the adenoids may then result in even greater nasal escape and hypernasal speech. Although the anatomical integrity of pharynx and larynx can be examined by an ENT surgeon using laryngeal mirrors, the nasopharynx and the base of the skull can now be visualized with great clarity using MRI (Fig. 2.8) as well as by per nasal endoscopy.

Neurological dysarthria

If there is a disorder of the muscles of articulation, the consonants will be imprecisely articulated, the speech will be slow, slurred and difficult to understand, the voice may be harsh and monotonous with no intonation, phrases are short, and speech comes in bursts

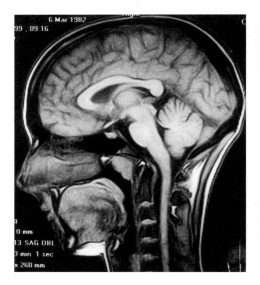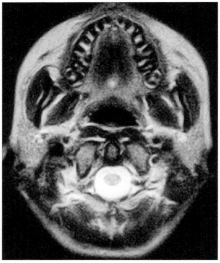

Fig. 2.8. MRI scans showing the brainstem, pons and medulla as well as the anatomy of lips, tongue, palate and larynx.

and shows excessive hyper- or hyponasality. Speaking is associated with increased effort and consciousness of the act of articulation, which is normally subconscious. Respiratory control is poor, so that a breath is taken in the middle of a word or phrase.

ANATOMY OF BULBAR FUNCTION

The same muscles used in articulation have additional important functions in feeding. Biting, chewing, swallowing, respiration, phonation and articulation share the same final pathway and muscles. Polygraphic studies of breathing looking at nasal airflow and its synchrony with chest movements, especially during sleep, along with overnight pulse oximetry, should form part of the routine investigation of brainstem function. At brainstem level specialization of function is already taking place in specialized nuclei, *e.g.* facial movement (facial nucleus), salivation (salivatory nucleus), mastication (masticatory nucleus), respiration (nucleus of tractus solitarius) and taste (gustatory nucleus) (Fig. 2.9).

Facial movements are represented in the large facial nuclei on each side of the midline in the upper part of the fourth ventricle. The face is particularly involved in emotional expression, but lip closure by the orbicularis oris is important in speech and feeding. Tongue movements are represented by the hypoglossal nucleus on each side of the midline in the bottom half of the fourth ventricle, and the tongue has its own nerve supply through the hypoglossal nerves. Closely related developmentally to these nuclei is the nucleus ambiguus which is responsible for the control of movement of the pharynx and larynx; neural impulses from the brainstem nuclei reach the muscles by the glossopharyngeal, accessory and vagus nerves. The nucleus ambiguus is unusual in that it supplies muscles of the larynx using

52

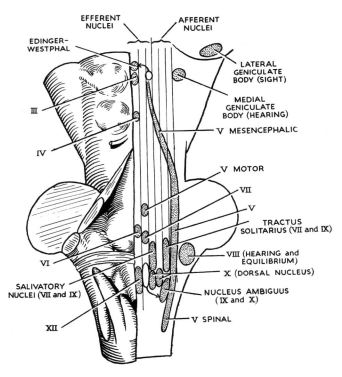

Fig. 2.9. Diagrammatic representation of the nuclei in the pons and medulla that control movement of the face, lips, tongue and palate as well as specialization for breathing, salivation, mastication and taste. The nuclei tend to remain in columns dependent on whether they are motor or sensory and whether voluntary or autonomic. (Reproduced by permission from Last 1956.)

parasympathetic fibres to supply striated muscle. Another motor nucleus, the vagal motor nucleus sends all of its motor impulses via the parasympathetic component of the Xth cranial (vagus) nerve and is responsible for oesophageal and gastric motility. There must obviously be close cooperation between the nucleus ambiguus and the dorsal vagal nucleus so that swallowing is a coordinated and continuous action; this can now be demonstrated dynamically using videofluoroscopy. If this cooperation is lacking then a functional block at the level of the cricopharyngeus can occur similar to that seen in achalasia at the lower end of the oesophagus.

Biting and chewing depend more on the powerful pincer effects resulting from contraction of the masseter, temporalis and pterygoid muscles. These muscles receive their motor supply separately via the motor division of the mandibular branch of the trigeminal nerve, and their central connection is to the masticatory nucleus and not the nucleus ambiguus. They may become spastic and are involved in the jaw jerk but, very importantly, are not involved in articulation. Sensation from the larynx, pharynx and gut is transmitted via the afferent fibres in the VIIth, IXth and Xth cranial nerves which go to the nucleus of the tractus

TABLE 2.2
Clinical aspects of bulbar function

Normal function	Abnormal function
Articulation	Imprecise consonants, slow, slurred, laboured
Phonation	Harsh voice, breathy, aphonia, monotone, loss of high frequencies
Airway protection	Asphyxiate aspirate, absent gag or cough
Mastication	Spastic jaw, no bite, no chew
Salvation	Drooling
Taste	Dysgeusia
Swallow	Dysphagia
Palatal closure of nasopharynx	Nasal escape, poor intrabuccal pressure, recurrent aspiration
Respiratory control	Inspire when swallowing and aspirate
Oral sensation	Anaesthesia, burns, mutilation

TABLE 2.3
Clinical and anatomical comparison of bulbar function

Bulbar function	Cranial nerve	Nucleus in the bulb
Tongue function	Hypoglossal	Hypoglossal nucleus
Pharyngeal movement	Hypoglossal	Nucleus ambiguus
	Glossopharyngeal	Nucleus ambiguus
Mastication	Trigeminal	Trigeminal nucleus
Lip closure	Facial	Facial nucleus (upper half of 4th ventricle floor)
Taste	Facial via chorda tympani	Tractus solitarius
	Glossopharyngeal	Tractus solitarius (lateral medulla above inferior cerebellar peduncle)
Touch	Trigeminal (lingual branch)	Trigeminal nucleus

solitarius. This latter nucleus is also involved in the control of breathing. Taste sensation is transmitted by the chorda tympani branch of the facial nerve. It can therefore be seen that mastication, salivation, taste, swallowing and articulation all share the same cranial nerves as a final common path; they have already been sorted into separate functions at brainstem level (Tables 2.2, 2.3). A lesion in a cranial nerve may cause a disorder localized to a particular anatomical segment, *e.g.* wasting of one side of the tongue or paralysis of half the soft palate. Each nucleus may make connections with other nuclei in the brainstem allowing development of the so-called brainstem reflexes. Three main groups of brainstem reflexes—protective, primitive and stretch reflexes—help to define the various types of bulbar palsy (Brown 1985) (Table 2.4).

PROTECTIVE REFLEXES
These reflexes protect: (1) the upper airway as in sneezing; (2) against aspiration and obstruction of the airway as with coughing and stridor; and (3) against ingestion of harmful material as with vomiting and the gag reflex.

TABLE 2.4
Comparison of the various types of bulbar dysfunction

Bulbar dysfunction	Protective reflexes	Primitive reflexes	Jaw tone	Jaw jerk	Face	Swallow dysphasia	Respiration, risk of aspiration	Dysarthria	Voluntary bite
Lower motor neuron	–	–	Hypotonic	–	Droopy	+++	++++	+++	–
Supranuclear bulbar palsy	++++	–	Spastic	++++	Fixed, immobile	+++	+	++++	Spastic bite ++ Voluntary –
Hyperkinetic bulbar palsy	++	++++	Rigidity fluctuates with position of head and contact	–	Grin	++	–	+++	+ or –
Hypokinetic bulbar palsy	++	+	Rigid	–	Sad, immobile	– or +	–	+ or ++	+ or –
Ataxic bulbar palsy	++	–	Hypotonic	++	Droopy, mouth open	– or +	–	+ Developmental pattern	++
Dyspraxia	++	–	Normal	++	Normal	–	–	Developmental or deviant	++

TABLE 2.5
The primitive feeding reflexes

Positive (ingesting)	Negative (avoidance reflexes)
Rooting reflex	Facial avoidance
Cardinal points reflex	Pursing lip rejection
Tonic mouth opening	Tongue rejection, impaction against roof of
Rhythmic, non-nutritive, sucking	mouth
Cricopharyngeal relaxation	Tongue rolling, 'adder tonguing' (rhythmic
	movements)
	Cricopharyngeal spasm
	Gagging
	Spastic bite

TABLE 2.6
Causes of a lower motor neuron, hypotonic 'true' bulbar palsy

Anterior horn cell disease	Neuromuscular junction
Werdnig–Hoffman disease	Neonatal myasthenia gravis
Fazio–Londe syndrome	Congenital myasthenia gravis
Von Laere syndrome	Juvenile myasthenia gravis
Motor neuron disease	Botulism
Porphyria	Diphtheria
Brainstem nuclei	**Peripheral nerve**
Neonatal asphyxia	Polyneuritis cranialis
Brainstem dysplasias	Leukaemia
Moebius syndrome	Sarcoidosis
Pontine glioma	Nasopharyngeal tumours
Rhombencephalitis	Juvenile Paget's disease
Dandy–Walker malformation	Osteopetrosis
Birth injury (vertebral artery, posterior	Zellweger syndrome
fossa haemorrhage)	Glomus jugulare tumours
Head injury	
Syringobulbia	**Muscle disease**
	Infant of mother with dystrophia myotonica
Metabolic disease	Mitochondrial myopathy
Malignant hyperphenylalaninemia	Nemaline myopathy
Propionic acidaemia	Myotubular myopathy
Leigh's encephalopathy	Oculopharyngeal dystrophy
Non-ketotic hyperglycinaemia	Central core disease
Infantile Gaucher disease	Whistling face syndrome

PRIMITIVE FEEDING REFLEXES
The various types of primitive feeding reflex are listed in Table 2.5.

True or lower motor neuron bulbar palsy
Included within this subgroup (Table 2.6) are all diseases that affect the lower motor neuron, *viz.* anterior horn cell, peripheral nerve, neuromuscular junction and the muscle itself. There may be involvement of all the muscles of mastication, swallowing and articulation, or of individual cranial nerves causing a more localized lesion. The muscles of the soft palate,

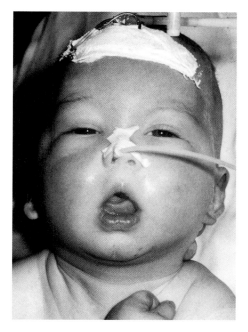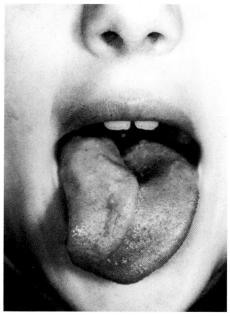

Fig. 2.10. Bilateral facial palsy with bulbar palsy affecting bite, chew, swallow and airway protection.

Fig. 2.11. Hemiatrophy of the tongue from hypoglossal paralysis.

pharynx and larynx are often the most obvious. In a lower motor neuron lesion, all functions of the muscle—voluntary, emotional and reflex—are lost. There is impaired biting, chewing and swallowing, drooling, aspiration of saliva and food, nasal reflux and speechlessness.

The clinical presentation of a flaccid bulbar palsy is a droopy face and a lax open mouth with jaw muscle atonia, and weakness and wasting of masseters and tongue (Fig. 2.10). There is drooling, feeding is difficult, the jaw and gag reflexes are absent, and there is no cough reflex. The absence of protective reflexes means that food may be aspirated into the lungs, and there is usually a severe dysarthria or anarthria. There are no primitive reflexes and no stretch reflexes. The tongue is wasted, will not protrude and shows fasciculation. Stridor can occur if the vocal cords are affected; the voice itself will be weak and breathy. The palate will not move with the gag reflex or upon saying "ah". If isolated cranial nerves are involved the tongue may only be wasted on the affected side and deviate on protrusion (Fig. 2.11), or alternatively, one-half of the palate may rise with the gag reflex and the uvula move to that side.

Many of the disorders that affect the lower motor neuron are progressive so that there may be clinical deterioration from mild dysarthria and drooling with tongue deviation, to a total anarthria, the need to tube feed and distressing accumulation of secretions leading to aspiration, pneumonia and death.

The bulbar muscles may be affected in the congenital form of myotonic dystrophy in which severe feeding problems present at birth, gradually improve, but are followed by slow speech development, which is aggravated by the associated learning disability. The Prader–Willi syndrome may present as congenital bulbar palsy with drooping, drooling facies and slow speech development associated with intellectual slowness. Bulbar muscle function will improve as the infant gets older in both of these conditions, so that normal feeding may eventually be possible. Myasthenia gravis in childhood may have an oculopharyngeal presentation and this can be acute, precipitated by a virus infection. The abnormal eye movements may be asymmetrical, as may palatal movements, and the condition may mimic a brainstem tumour.

A complete bulbar palsy will necessitate long-term tube feeding or gastrostomy, and is associated with a persisting anarthria necessitating an augmented communication system. Tracheotomy may be essential for suctioning if recurrent aspiration of saliva or gastric contents threatens life. The disastrous prognosis of these conditions means that onset of dysarthria in a child must always be taken as an indication for a full and detailed neurological examination.

Pseudobulbar palsy (spastic dysarthria)
This is an upper motor neuron type of bulbar palsy with release of the brainstem reflexes from cortical and midbrain control. The jaw is stiff, the mouth is difficult to open fully, and the jaw jerk is brisk and often accompanied by jaw clonus. The tongue is small and bunched, and rapid movements such as protruding and moving from side to side are difficult, although some movement of the tongue is usually possible. Biting and chewing are difficult due to the spastic masseter muscles. There is no wasting, for example of the temporalis muscle. The protective reflexes are present, the gag reflex is very brisk, the cough reflex is present, and inhalation is less common than in bulbar palsy as the airway retains its reflex protection. Drooling is often a problem.

Speech, if there is any, is slow and laboured with poor variation in pitch; it is hypernasal, the voice is harsh, and the rhythm may be explosive. Consonants are imprecise and slurred; emphasis is absent or is applied in the wrong place. The child finds it difficult to control breathing for speech, thus interfering with normal phrasing.

Speech remains difficult to interpret even in adults with cerebral palsy, only half of whose utterances may be understood by strangers, speech being more difficult to understand in athetosis than in spastic cerebral palsy. The pattern of poor anterior tongue placement, difficulty with fricatives and slower speech is preserved from childhood to the adult (Platt *et al.* 1980a,b).

MUSCLE STRETCH REFLEXES
The jaw jerk is a simple monosynaptic reflex through the temporalis and masseter muscles in which tapping the semi-opened jaw on the chin results in a brisk contraction or, if the reflex is uninhibited, jaw clonus. In severely brain damaged individuals with brainstem release, tapping the lips causes reflex pursing due to tonic contraction of the orbicularis oris. In order for these reflexes to be present the muscle and cranial nerve must be connected via the nucleus to the sensory supply from the muscle spindles to the masticatory nucleus.

The bulbar muscles involved in speech have bilateral cortical representation so that although a unilateral cortical lesion can cause speech dyspraxia or expressive aphasia, a bilateral lesion is necessary to cause a pseudobulbar palsy. This is seen in opercular dysplasia and the late syndrome of herpes simplex encephalitis (see below). Dysarthria/anarthria is not therefore seen with hemiplegia but is the rule with tetraplegia.

The commonest causes of pseudobulbar palsy seen in childhood are associated with cerebral palsy, especially following perinatal asphyxia. Any other severe hypoxic–ischaemic episode such as may result from uncontrolled status epilepticus, drowning, poisoning, cardiac arrest, etc. may cause a pseudobulbar palsy. Encephalitis and brainstem tumours may cause a mixed upper and lower motor neuron picture, as may amyotrophic lateral sclerosis. Another common cause of pseudobulbar palsy in children is head injury with mid-brain or upper brainstem damage associated with deceleration or acceleration and secondary brainstem ischaemia due to tentorial herniation causing impairment of the vascular supply to the central parts of the brainstem and consequent secondary haemorrhage. Dysarthria can be extremely severe after a head injury in children but speech recovery may be good.

Multiple sclerosis, which is a common cause of pseudobulbar palsy and dysarthria in adolescents and young adults, is not common in prepubertal children.

An acquired bulbar palsy has a much more sinister prognosis than a congenital pseudo-bulbar palsy, which is usually associated with nonprogressive cerebral palsy. Degenerative brain diseases not uncommonly present with dysarthria and a spastic pseudobulbar palsy, especially conditions such as subacute sclerosing encephalitis, metachromatic leukodystrophy, Alexander's disease, Batten's disease and the adolescent form of GM2 gangliosidosis.

There is a relatively unusual form of isolated pseudobulbar palsy, described initially by Worster Drought, that may present in early infancy with feeding difficulties and has long-lasting effects on speech. There is then delay in speech development with dysarthria accompanied by drooling, poor control of fast tongue movements, poor palatal movements and a very brisk jaw jerk, but little feeding difficulty by the time the child is 3 or 4 years of age, although still marked difficulty with speech. There may be brisk tendon reflexes and extensor plantar reflexes. MRI may show an opercular dysplasia. This occurs without any obvious cause, and must be differentiated from bulbar weakness secondary to perinatal asphyxia and the similar syndrome as a late consequence of herpes simplex encephalitis. The condition is often known as the bilateral perisylvian syndrome and is thought to be a developmental, probably genetically determined condition.

Extrapyramidal or dyskinetic dysarthria
Dyskinetic bulbar palsies have been divided into two forms, a hypokinetic and a hyperkinetic form.

The *hypokinetic* form is seen most commonly in parkinsonism and only seldom in children. There are several causes in children, such as drugs, including haloperidol and valproate. There is a congenital metabolic failure of dopamine synthesis, and certain types of genetic dystonia in childhood, *e.g.* Segawa disease, may develop into parkinsonism in adolescence. Parkinsonism is also seen in subacute encephalitis, encephalitis lethargica and Batten's disease.

The face is expressionless, the voice slow, monotonous, of little volume and sometimes accompanied by festination of speech, *i.e.* mainly a loss of the prosodic aspects of speech involving intonation and cadence (see pp. 29–30).

Hyperkinetic bulbar palsy is much more common in children. Many unwanted movements interfere with normal articulation. These movements are both reflex and involuntary in type and are seen in association with choreoathetosis that affects limb and trunk muscles. The hallmark of hyperkinetic bulbar palsy as opposed to a pseudobulbar palsy is the obligatory retention in the former of all the infant feeding reflexes, so that rooting, reflex bite, cardinal points, lip reflexes, sucking and tonic mouth opening are all easily elicited. Tonic opening of the mouth, which the child cannot overcome, occurs if the head is extended and traction applied to the hands (palmomental reflex) or if the perioral region is stimulated with a metal spoon. It also forms part of a mass extensor response to a sudden shock or anxiety.

The tongue is often protruded in a tonic manner or may show rolling rhythmic movements ('adder tonguing'). The gag reflexes, cough reflexes and all protective reflexes are retained so that aspiration of food in early childhood is uncommon, as the airway remains protected, but this may change with ageing. The jaw jerk is present but not exaggerated unless there is a mixed lesion, as in spastic dyskinesia. Chewing and biting are difficult, feeding is messy and particular care must be taken not to trigger the various reflexes. Saliva control is often poor.

In children with hyperkinetic bulbar palsy, speech is difficult to understand and is associated with a lot of grimacing and torsion movements of the head and limbs. It is often very explosive and slurred, and coming in rushes sometimes on an ingressive air stream. The pitch is monotonous, volume is uncontrolled, voice quality can be harsh, and both vowels and consonants may be distorted. Intelligence may be well preserved. This condition includes one of the most important groups of children, in whom learning disability may be wrongly diagnosed in early childhood due to severe communication difficulties. These severely anarthric children are helped considerably by alternative communication systems. In children with postkernicteric hyperkinetic bulbar palsy, although intelligence is preserved, the condition can be aggravated by an associated sensorineural deafness.

As the child gets older, lips, tongue and palate will become progressively more involved in involuntary movements so that grimacing, chewing movements, tongue rolling, clucking and pharyngeal movements become more obvious. These are seen in their manifest form in the isolated, so-called orofacial dyskinesias and tardive dyskinesias, which may follow prolonged use of phenothiazine drugs, especially haloperidol.

Causes of hyperkinetic bulbar palsy

Kernicterus, which used to be the commonest cause of a pure extrapyramidal syndrome in childhood, is now rare but is still seen in the Far East from glucose-6-phosphate dehydrogenase deficiency. More mixed spastic/dyskinetic patterns following perinatal asphyxia are commoner. Severe hypoxia, as from carbon monoxide poisoning, uncontrolled status epilepticus, or cardiac bypass surgery, may result in dyskinetic bulbar paresis with an associated marked dysarthria. There is a group of metabolic degenerative diseases that can

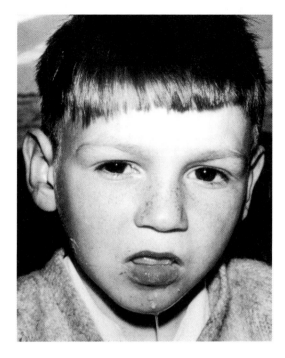

Fig. 2.12. Eversion of lower lip, flattened nasolabial creases and severe drooling in a boy with ataxic bulbar palsy.

also selectively affect the basal ganglia, as seen for example in Fahr syndrome, mitochondrial encephalopathies, Leigh's encephalopathy, glutaric aciduria, Hallervorden–Spatz disease, heavy metal poisoning, etc.

Ataxic bulbar palsy
In ataxic bulbar palsies the face is hypotonic and droopy, the mouth open, and drooling may be marked (Fig. 2.12). Superficially it resembles a lower motor neuron bulbar palsy, but bite, chew and swallow are preserved, protective reflexes are normal and jaw jerk is present.

Children with acquired destructive lesions of the cerebellum such as occur with cerebellar tumours like astrocytoma or haemangioblastoma, or cerebellar degenerations, may develop ataxic dysarthria. Disorders such as Friedreich's ataxia with gross incoordination of limbs and trunk are associated with a gross dysarthria but not usually until the later teens, while other causes of degenerative ataxia such as ataxia–telangiectasia may have an early dysarthric component. In these cases the force, speed and distance for precise muscle movement as described above are disrupted so speech varies in volume, is explosive and slurred, varies from phrase to phrase and is often staccato.

Children with ataxia from infancy due to hydrocephalus, cerebellar hypoplasia, vermis aplasia, perinatal asphyxia, hypothyroidism or the various genetic syndromes have a developmental pattern of delayed articulation, *i.e.* a delay in motor learning. As speech develops there may be features of ataxic dysarthria, and possible dyspraxias.

Summary

In this and the previous chapter we have attempted to demonstrate the neural pathways involved in inner language and speech as a continuum so that the clinician can approach the child with some sort of schema for history, examination and investigation.

Prior to augmenting communication, an accurate assessment and diagnosis of the communication disorder must be made. After a careful history and clinical examination, a full speech and language assessment will be required in order to make an overall clinical diagnosis. More specific investigations may then be required: these may include audiometric techniques from free field testing to electrocochleography and cortical evoked responses. Imaging of the brain for gross anatomical lesions and functional imaging using SPECT, PET and functional MRI will become more important and routine in the future. Chromosome analysis including DNA testing for fragile X is indicated in all cases of learning disability and receptive dysphasia. Again in the future, as more genetic syndromes are recognized and we have cytogenetic localization, we will be able to diagnose specific genetic diseases, *e.g.* articulatory dyspraxia, receptive aphasia and some cases of dyslexia on more specific DNA tests. A case can be made for all cases of dysarthria with severe bulbar palsy being investigated anatomically by MRI and videofluoroscopy. In specific cases differential airflow studies between nose and mouth, spectrographic analysis of speech, and palatal examination by pernasal endoscopy may be helpful.

REFERENCES

Abraham, S.S., Wallace, I.F., Gravel, J.S. (1996) 'Early otitis media and phonological development at age 2 years.' *Laryngoscope*, **106**, 727–732.

Bishop, D.V. (1980) 'Handedness, clumsiness and cognitive ability.' *Developmental Medicine and Child Neurology*, **22**, 569–579.

—— (1997) 'Pre- and perinatal hazards and family background in children with specific language impairments: a study of twins.' *Brain and Language*, **56**, 1–26.

Bouchard, S., Lallier, M., Yazbeck, S., Bensoussan, A. (1999) 'The otolaryngologic manifestations of gastro-esophageal reflux: when is a pH study indicated?' *Journal of Pediatric Surgery*, **6**, 1053–1056.

Brown, J.K. (1969) 'Feeding reflexes in infancy.' *Developmental Medicine and Child Neurology*, **11**, 641.

—— (1985) 'Dysarthria in children: neurological perspective.' *In: Speech and Language Evaluation in Neurology*. New York: Grune & Stratton, pp. 133–184.

—— Minns, R. (1999)' The neurological basis of learning disorders in children.' *In:* Whitmore, K., Hart, H., Willems, G. (Eds.) *A Neurodevelopmental Approach to Specific Learning Disorders. Clinics in Developmental Medicine No. 145*. London: Mac Keith Press, pp. 24–75.

Burden, V., Stott, C.M., Forge, J., Goodyer, I. (1996) 'The Cambridge Language and Speech Project (CLASP). I. Detection of language difficulties at 36 to 39 months.' *Developmental Medicine and Child Neurology*, **38**, 613–631.

Butler, N., Sheridan, M.D., Peckham, C. (1973) 'Speech defects in children.' *British Medical Journal*, **2**, 780–781.

Catsman-Berrevoets, C.E., Van Dongen, H.R. (1997) 'The syndrome of cerebellar mutism and subsequent dysarthria: incidence and pathophysiology.' *European Journal of Paediatric Neurology*, **1**, A32–A33.

—— —— Mulder, P.G., y Geuze, D.P., Paquier, P.F., Lequin, M.H. (1999) 'Tumour type and size are high risk factors for syndrome of "cerebellar" mutism and subsequent dysarthria.' *Journal of Neurology, Neurosurgery and Psychiatry*, **67**, 755–757.

Elbert, T., Pantev, C., Wienbruch, C., Rockstroh, B., Taub, E. (1995) 'Increased cortical representation of the fingers of the left hand in string players.' *Science*, **270**, 305–307.

Ferlito, A., Rinaldo, A., Marioni, G. (1999) 'Laryngeal malignant neoplasms in children and adolescents.' *International Journal of Pediatric Otorhinolaryngology*, **49**, 1–14.

Fisher, S., Vargha-Khadem, F., Watkins, K.E, Monaco, A.P., Pembry, M.E. (1998) 'Localization of a gene implicated in a severe speech and language disorder.' *Nature Genetics*, **18**, 168–170.

Galaburda, A.M. (1999) 'Albert Einstein's brain.' *Lancet*, **354**, 1821. *(Letter.)*

Germano, A., Baldari, S., Caruso, G., Caffo, G., Montemango, G., Gardia, E., Tomasello, F. (1998) 'Reversible cerebral perfusion alteration in children with transient mutism after posterior fossa surgery.' *Child's Nervous System*, **14**, 114–119.

Ghazala, Q.R. (1993) 'Incantors – Circuit-bending and living instruments.' *Experimental Musical Instruments*, **8** (6), 18–21.

Ingram, T.T.S. (1959) 'Specific developmental disorders of speech in childhood.' *Brain*, **82**, 450–467.

—— (1972) 'Speech disorders in childhood.' *Proceedings of the Royal Society of Medicine*, **65**, 404–409.

—— (1973) 'The prevalence of speech disorders in childhood.' *Developmental Medicine and Child Neurology*, **15**, 656–658.

Jackson, L.D., Polygenis, D., McIvor, R.A., Worthington, I. (1999) 'Comparative efficacy and safety of inhaled corticosteroids in asthma.' *Canadian Journal of Clinical Pharmacology*, **6**, 26–37.

Kornse, D.D., Manni, J.L., Rubenstein, H., Graziani, L.J. (1981) 'Developmental apraxia of speech and manual dexterity.' *Journal of Communication Disorders*, **14**, 321–330.

Last, R.J. (1956) *Anatomy, Regional and Applied.* London: J. & A. Churchill.

Lewis, B.A., Freebairn, L. (1998) 'Speech production skills of nuclear family members of children with phonological disorders.' *Language and Speech*, **41**, 45–61.

Loganovskaja, T.K., Loganovsky, K.N. (1999) 'EEG, cognitive and psychopathology abnormalities in children irradiated *in utero*.' *International Journal of Psychophysiology*, **34**, 213–224.

Lou, H.C., Henricksen, L.., Bruhn, P. (1984) 'Focal cerebral hypoperfusion in children with dysphasia and/or attention deficit disorder.' *Archives of Neurology*, **41**, 825–829.

Maw, A.R. (1995) *Glue Ear in Childhood. Clinics in Developmental Medicine No. 135.* London: Mac Keith Press.

McMackin, D., Jones-Gotman, M., Dubeau, F., Gotman, J., Lukban, A., Dean, G., Evans, A., Lisbonna, R. (1998) 'Regional cerebral blood flow and language dominance: SPECT during intracarotid amobarbital testing.' *Neurology*, **50**, 943–950.

McNeill, D. (1970) *The Acquisition of Language.* New York: Harper & Row.

Mohr, J.P., Pessin, M.S., Finkelstein, S., Funkenstein, H.H., Duncan, G.W., Davis, K.R. (1978) 'Broca aphasia: pathologic and clinical.' *Neurology*, **28**, 311–324.

Naeser, M.A., Palumbo, C.L., Helm-Estabrooks, N., Stiassny-Eder, D., Albert, M.L. (1989) 'Severe non-fluency in apahasia: role of the medial subcallosal fasciculus and other white matter pathways in the recovery of spontaneous speech.' *Brain*, **112**, 1–38.

O'Hare, A.E., Brown, J.K. (1997) 'Speech and language disorders in disorders of the central nervous system.' *In:* Campbell, A.G.M., McIntosh, N. (Eds.) *Forfar and Arneil's Textbook of Paediatrics, 5th Edn.* Edinburgh: Churchill Livingstone, pp. 804–818.

O'Regan, M.E., Brown, J.K., Goodwin, G.M., Clarke, M. (1998) 'Epileptic aphasia: a consequence of regional hypometabolic encephalopathy.' *Developmental Medicine and Child Neurology*, **40**, 508–517.

Owen, S.E., McKinlay, I.A. (1997) 'Motor difficulties in children with developmental disorders of speech and language.' *Child: Care, Health and Development*, **23**, 315–325.

Paget, R. (1930) *Human Speech.* London: Harcourt Brace.

Petersen, S.E., Fox, P.T., Posner, M.I., Mitnum, M., Raichle, M.E. (1988) 'Positron emission tomographic studies of the cortical anatomy of single word processing.' *Nature*, **331**, 585–589.

Platt, L.J., Andrews, G., Howie, P.M. (1980a) 'Dysarthria of adult cerebral palsy. 2. Phonemic analysis of articulation errors.' *Journal of Speech and Hearing Research*, **23**, 41–55.

—————— Young, M., Quinn, P.T. (1980b) 'Dysarthria of adult cerebral palsy. 1. Intelligibility and articulatory impairment.' *Journal of Speech and Hearing Research*, **23**, 28–40.

Rapin, I. (1996) *Preschool Children with Inadequate Communication. Clinics in Developmental Medicine No. 139.* London: Mac Keith Press.

Reid, L., Rumsey, J.M., Nace, K., Andreason, J.M. (1996) *Neuroimaging: A Window to the Neurological Foundations of Learning and Behaviour in Children.* Baltimore: Paul H. Brookes.

Robinson, R. (1991) 'Causes and associations of severe and persistent specific speech and language disorders in children.' *Developmental Medicine and Child Neurology*, **33**, 943–962.

Scheffer, I.E., Jones, L., Pozzebon, M., Howell, R.A., Saling, M.M., Berkovic, S.F. (1995) 'Autosomal dominant rolandic epilepsy and speech dyspraxia: a new syndrome with anticipation.' *Annals of Neurology*, **38**: 633–642.

Silva, P.A. (1980) 'A study of the prevalence, stability and significance of developmental language delays in preschool children.' *Developmental Medicine and Child Neurology*, **22**, 768–777.

—— McGee, R., Williams, S.M. (1983) 'Developmental language delay from three to seven years and its significance for low intelligence and reading difficulties at age seven.' *Developmental Medicine and Child Neurology*, **25**, 783–793.

Stevenson, J., Richman, N. (1976) 'The prevalence of language delay in a population of three year old children.' Journal of Autism and Childhood Schizophrenia, **8**, 299–313.

Stothard, S.E., Snowling, M.J., Bishop, D.V., Chipchase, B.B., Kaplan, C.A. (1998) 'Language impaired preschoolers: a follow up into adolescence.' *Journal of Speech, Language and Hearing Research*, **41**, 407–418.

Templin, M.C. (1957) *Certain Language Skills in Children, their Developmental and Interrelationships. Institute of Child Welfare, Monograph No. 26.* Minneapolis: University of Minnesota Press.

Van Borsel, J. (1988) 'An analysis of the speech of five Down's syndrome adolescents.' *Journal of Communication Disorders*, **21**, 409–421.

Van Hout, A., Evrard, P., Lyon, G. (1985) 'On the positive seminology of acquired aphasia in children.' *Developmental Medicine and Child Neurology*, **27**, 231–241.

Vargha-Khadem, F., Watkins, K.E., Price, C.J., Ashburner, J., Alcock, K.J., Connelly, A., Frackowiak, R.S., Friston, K.J., Mishkin, M., *et al.* (1998) 'Neural basis of inherited speech and language disorder.' *Proceedings of the National Academy of Sciences of the USA*, **95**, 12695–12700.

Wada, J., Rasmussen, T. (1960) 'Intracarotid injection of sodium amytal for the lateralization of cerebral speech dominance.' *Journal of Neurosurgery*, **17**, 266–282.

Wise, R.J., Greene, J., Buchel, C., Scott, S.K. (1999) 'Brain regions involved in articulation.' *Lancet*, **353**, 1057–1061.

Witelson, D.F. (1976) 'Sex and the single hemisphere: specialization of the right hemisphere for spatial processing.' *Science*, **193**, 425–427.

3
WHO NEEDS AUGMENTATIVE AND ALTERNATIVE COMMUNICATION, AND WHEN?

Martin Bax, Helen Cockerill, Lesley Carroll-Few

Many children are at risk of having a speech and language impairment, as a result of which they may require the use of AAC systems. Most families are extremely keen that their child should develop the traditional oral mode of communication and are often somewhat reluctant to recognize that this may prove very difficult for the child to achieve. The paediatrician's role in this instance is to try to help the family achieve a realistic view of what is possible for the child and what is not. There are various groups of children who are likely to have such problems.

Cerebral palsy
The rate of cerebral palsy in the developed world is between 2 and 2.5 per 1000 (Stanley *et al*. 2000). However, there are few available epidemiological data on the rates of speech and language problems in children with cerebral palsy. The older, large studies of cerebral palsy by Crothers and Paine (1959) and Ingram (1964) probably present as much useful data as many later studies where good language/communication data are often not reported. Ingram (whose study, based on children in the east of Scotland, has a sounder epidemiological basis than that of Crothers and Paine) reported that nearly half of his patients (102 of 208) had "defective articulation". He noted the high rate of problems in dyskinetic patients. He found more difficulty in assessing language development because of the presence of learning difficulties but noted that the "degree of language difficulty was out of all proportion to the severity of the mental retardation".

Crothers and Paine, reporting a sample derived from their patients attending the Washington Children's Hospital, also drew attention to the high rates of speech and language problems. These were especially prevalent in children with hemiplegia: 34 of the 82 children with congenital hemiplegia and 34 of 47 with acquired hemiplegia had speech problems. Of 127 children with athetosis 98 had speech problems. In children with tetraplegia speech and language problems correlated with intelligence, which of course was not the case in those with athetosis.

However, the current proportion of children with this disorder who are going to require AAC is unknown. The Family Fund Trust, based at the Social Policy Research Unit of the University of York, holds the largest database of children with severe disabilities in the UK (self-selected population); among those with cerebral palsy around half have feeding difficulties (unpublished data). Children with feeding (oromotor) difficulties commonly have speech problems. In a survey of 18- to 25-year-olds based on a whole population of people with moderate to severe motor disabilities, over half the 45 young adults with cerebral palsy had moderate or severe communication problems (Thomas *et al.* 1989). In an ongoing European multicentre population-based study of 2-year-old children with cerebral palsy, 60 per cent are recorded as having a communication problem after examination by a paediatrician (M. Bax and C. Tydeman, unpublished data).

All children with cerebral palsy may have speech problems, but those with athetoid cerebral palsy have particularly high rates. A survey by Foley (1983) of 165 indicated that 63 per cent were without speech at the age of 5 years. Children with pure athetosis may have reasonable cognitive ability but severe dysarthria. The group with spastic quadriplegia have very high rates of communication problems. Learning difficulties are present in a high proportion, and consequently their speech difficulties are compounded by cognitive factors. In the less severely affected children with spastic diplegia and hemiplegia, problems with language or speech may be present. It is possible to see in a child with diplegia or hemiplegia a very clear articulatory dyspraxia. However, in children with hemiplegia language is usually preserved (Mutter and Vargha-Khadem 2000), although speech may not be (Crothers and Paine 1959).

Spina bifida

In the other most common physical disability, namely spina bifida, speech and language problems are also common (Thomas *et al.* 1989). These are most likely to occur in those children who have additional hydrocephalus. In the same population study referred to above, a third of the young people had some problems with communication. This serves to emphasize that attention must be paid to the communication problems of all young children with a physical disability and that consideration of the possible role of AAC in supporting communication should be made.

Learning disabilities

Learning disability, or mental retardation, is a blanket term for a wide variety of genetic, social and specific medical conditions that share the common feature of a score below 70 on IQ tests. Approximately 6 per 1000 of the population have a moderate to severe learning disorder. Insofar as cognitive ability plays a prominent part in the acquisition of language, it is inevitable that virtually all these children will have some disorder of communication. Children with Down syndrome in the highest ability range will have restricted vocabularies and sentence structures. Where the cognitive level is over 60 usually some level of oral speech and language is achieved. As the IQ deficit becomes more severe the chances of a language problem are increased. It is interesting to note that babies with Down syndrome have abnormal and prolonged cries, but their eventual level of speech, if acquired, is not noticeably dysarthric. However, voice quality is often distinctive.

Many syndromes that include a learning disability are associated with some form of disorder of tone. As a consequence, difficulties may be encountered with articulation. A proportion may have a severe articulation impairment or a verbal dyspraxia.

Syndromes

A variety of syndromes involve specific speech impairments, often in conjunction with a degree of learning disability. These include Moebius syndrome, Treacher–Collins syndrome, congenital bilateral perisylvian (Worster Drought) syndrome and 22q deletion or velocardio-facial syndrome.

Hearing impairment

The problems of children with moderate to profound hearing loss are well described. Where the child does not have additional motor problems, signing systems are obviously appropriate. The long-running debate about oralism—the notion that the child should not be taught sign language because this would discourage use of an oral system—is hopefully in the past because it is now well established that a signing system actually encourages the development of the oral system rather than in any way preventing it. There are syndromes of sensorineural deafness that are associated with learning disabilities, and equally the other conditions discussed in this review may be associated with a hearing deficit, for example cerebral palsy. In addition, there are particular groups of children with hearing problems who present additional visual impairment.

Autism

AAC may play a role in the attempt to establish communication in autism. The high-functioning autistic child and the child with Asperger syndrome will usually develop spoken language, although this may be used in a very idiosyncratic manner. Approximately 50 per cent of children with autism have learning difficulties, and some of these will not develop speech. Children with autism process visual information more effectively than auditory information, therefore many educational approaches use pictorial materials to support language comprehension, even with children who have developed speech, *e.g.* the TEACCH approach (Mesibov *et al.* 1984). For non-speaking autistic children picture symbols are increasingly used as a means of expression, teaching them to exchange pictures for desired objects and events (Bondy and Frost 1994). Visually based teaching and communication systems are being recognized as supplementing more traditional behavioural programmes where intervention is focused on teaching speech through imitation.

For an overview of approaches to communication in autism, see Trevarthen *et al.* (1996) and Howlin (1998).

Developmental speech and language disorders

The features of these conditions are difficult to determine due to the differences in criteria employed by different studies. It is usually thought that around 10 per cent of 3-year-old children (Bax *et al.* 1990) have speech and language that are significantly delayed. By the age of 5 the number of children identified with a significant problem is about 1 per cent, with a further 4 per cent exhibiting slight delay.

Children with developmental speech and language disorders fall into four main groups: expressive language disorders (aphasia); receptive–expressive disorders (receptive aphasia); phonological or sound system disorders; and stammering. Children in the last two groups are unlikely to benefit from AAC, but it may have a role in supporting language comprehension and expression in the first two.

Within the group of children with expressive disorders, certain specific speech impairments emerge—the dysarthrias and the dyspraxias. Dysarthria is where the speech production mechanism is impaired, with weak, inaccurate oral motor movements, although theoretically the child may have intact language. The disorder is rare in children with no other neurological impairments, although it may be a part of specific syndromes, *e.g.* congential bilateral perisylvian syndrome, where other neurological signs are minimal.

Dyspraxia (or developmental apraxia of speech) is where the tongue, lips and palate move appropriately for non-speech functions, but the coding by the brain of the accurate sequences of movements required to produce speech is impaired. In this group of children AAC has a role in facilitating communication alongside therapy aimed at developing speech production.

Cleft lip and palate and other structural disorders
Cleft lip and palate can be associated with articulatory problems, and AAC, usually manual signing systems, may play a role particularly at an early age while speech is developing. AAC is increasingly being used during temporary periods of speechlessness, on paediatric intensive care units, such as in facio-maxillary surgery (Costello 2000).

Epilepsy
There are a number of epileptic conditions in which speech and language may be affected. The best known is the Landau–Kleffner syndrome (Landau and Kleffner 1957). Here the child may have normal speech and language before the onset of epilepsy, but the epilepsy is associated with a loss of communication skills; in some cases these may subsequently be recovered (Mantovani and Landau 1980). Manual signing systems have been used with this population to support comprehension of spoken language and provide a means of expression (Vance 1991).

Acquired neurological conditions
Children who have CNS lesions due to traumatic brain injury (*e.g.* road traffic accidents, non-accidental injuries), tumours, stroke, etc., may demonstrate acquired aphasias, *i.e.* impairments to aspects of speech and language functioning. In this group of conditions AAC may have either a temporary or a permanent role, depending on the degree of recovery. It might be assumed that the majority of these children will have had normal pre-morbid language skills; however, it has been suggested that children with attention deficit hyperactivity disorder (ADHD) are at higher risk of traumatic brain injury (TBI), so that in some TBI patients who have ADHD, their speech/language disturbance may have been pre-existing.

Degenerative disorders
In many of these conditions, which are usually genetic, speech and language may be acquired and subsequently lost, often alongside physical and/or cognitive deterioration. There are

no available research data demonstrating efficacy of AAC in these conditions, but personal experience has demonstrated its value.

Possible roles of augmentative and alternative communication

In all of the conditions hitherto mentioned consideration must be given to the aims of introducing an AAC system. AAC can have a number of roles in facilitating communication.

- AAC can be used as an input system, to support comprehension of spoken language. By producing manual signs that correspond to the main words in a spoken message an adult speaker may attract a child's attention, the speech rate will be slowed, keywords will be emphasized and the child will be provided with additional visual information. Many signs have more direct relationship to the object or action represented than do spoken words (hence the increased use of gesture and mime when communicating with foreign language speakers). Similarly, pictures or symbols may be more easily recognized than auditory signals. Showing a child a visual stimulus while speaking may help to establish joint attention, and make meaning less ambiguous.
- The more established use of AAC is as an output system for children with limited or no speech.
- Computers and electronic communication aids can produce spoken and/or written output. The latter function is important for children with motor difficulties.
- Picture-based systems can provide a bridge to literacy in children with limited speech.

Paediatric assessment of the child who may need AAC

Paediatricians seeing children with disabilities use an age-related assessment process to look at the neurodevelopmental aspects of the child's condition. First the overall gross motor ability of the child would be considered, since gross motor competence and postural mechanisms impact on speech production. For example, breath control for speech production can be affected by truncal instability. Next the anatomical structures involved in speech would be examined. The speech apparatus—lungs, larynx, tongue, lips and palate—may have anatomical abnormalities, as for example in cleft lip and palate.

Hearing will be formally tested, and the ears and drums inspected. Middle ear disease is very common in children, but is commoner still in children with disabilities, with obvious implications for language development.

Feeding, saliva control and speech are related functions, but each can show disorder on its own. Historically it was believed that good feeding patterns laid the foundations for speech. However, the relationship between these functions is not clear. Netsell (1991) hypothesized that inhibition of the vegetative synapses is necessary for speech to be possible. It would seem that most children who do not progress beyond the suck–swallow pattern, who do not develop chewing or lateral tongue movements and who exhibit jaw hyperextension are likely to be children with concomitant severe speech impairment.

Observation of the child in interaction with her/his family in the assessment situation will yield valuable information with regard to social interaction and communicative intent.

The paediatrician will take a detailed case history from the caregivers, attempting to establish the child's level of understanding and ability to express her/himself. The development of vowel sounds (normally heard in early infancy), consonantal sounds (from around the age of 6 months), the first naming words (from 10 months onwards) and a rapidly growing vocabulary (beginning around 15–16 months) will all be considered in relation to the age of the child. Formal tests such as the Griffiths or Bailey scales may be of little value in children with disabilities.

Many clinicians, particularly when seeing children with disabilities who may have visual and motor problems, use informal methods to assess to what extent the child's expressive and receptive language are developing. The use of play materials, common objects, pictures, etc., is usual practice.

Once speech, language or communication problems have been identified most paediatricians will be assessing the child with the assistance of a specialist speech and language therapist and other professionals. More detailed and formal assessments can then be used (see Chapter 4). At this point many children with complex needs will be referred to specialist teams with additional skill in AAC.

Augmentative systems of communication include pictures, signs, symbols and technology, all of which are described in detail in subsequent chapters. The choice of system will depend on a range of factors such as the age, cognitive ability and physical skills of the child, and the ability of the child's caregivers and environment to support AAC. Parental expectations may veer towards the high-tech, but for young children low-tech systems are often more successful (Blackstone 1999).

In the typically developing child the majority of speech development will have taken place by the age of 5 years, with no intervention. However, in the group of children discussed in this chapter no predictable developmental pathway can be assumed. These children should be considered as potential users of AAC as soon as concerns about their future speech and language development are raised. The 'wait and see if speech develops' approach is no longer acceptable.

Discussion of the risk of speechlessness with the parents

Parents may often find it difficult to accept that their child may not be able to communicate with speech. The paediatrician is important in conveying to the parents the need that their child has for self-expression prior to any possible speech development. The focus of discussion should be on the development of communication rather than of speech alone. There are few published data on the impact of AAC on speech development. Whilst there is no shortage of anecdotal descriptions of the improvement in children's communication skills following the introduction of AAC, systematic documentation of the effects of AAC intervention on speech development is scarce. Millar *et al.* (2000) conducted a meta-analysis of 25 published studies on AAC intervention that included documentation of speech production, and concluded that there was no evidence of a negative effect on natural speech. While there was evidence of either an increase or no change in speech production in most of the studies analysed, the reported gains were minimal. Some recent AAC intervention studies have included specific data on speech production (*e.g.* Rowland and Schweigert 2000), but there is clearly a need for better evidence on this question.

Parents should be presented with clear information about the risk of speechlessness, with a realistic discussion about the limitations of oral motor therapy aimed at improving speech production. Again the literature on the effectiveness of articulation therapy on speech production in children is severely limited (Coombes 1984). Chinnery (2000), in a small-scale study of four children with athetoid cerebral palsy, was unable to demonstrate any change in intelligibility, despite minimal improvement in some speech production skills, in response to direct treatment of dysarthria.

Clinical experience suggests that an early focus on basic interaction skills and receptive language, with the gradual introduction of AAC strategies, within a family-centred model of service delivery is required for children who are at risk of failing to develop speech. Children who require AAC must have their needs for an expressive system met as early as possible if their language development is not to be further compromised.

REFERENCES

Bax, M., Hart, H., Jenkins, S.M. (1990) *Child Development and Child Health.* Oxford: Blackwell Scientific.

Blackstone, S. (1999) 'AAC approaches for infants and toddlers.' *Augmentative Communication News*, **12** (6), 2.

Bondy, A.S., Frost, LA.. (1994) 'The Picture Exchange Communication System.' *Focus on Autistic Behaviour*, **9**, 1–19.

Chinnery, C.L. (2000) 'Treatment effects on speech production and speech intelligibility of dysarthric speech in children with cerebral palsy.' MSc thesis, City University, London.

Coombes, K. (1984) 'Speech therapy.' *In:* Yule, W., Rutter, M. (Eds.) *Language Development and Disorders. Clinics in Developmental Medicine No. 101/102.* London: Mac Keith Press, pp. 350–366.

Costello, J.M. (2000) 'AAC intervention in the intensive care unit: the Children's Hospital Boston Model.' *Augmentative and Alternative Communication*, **16**, 137–153.

Crothers, B., Paine, R.S. (1959) *The Natural History of Cerebral Palsy.* Cambridge, MA: Harvard University Press. (Reprinted 1988 as *Classics in Developmental Medicine No. 2.* London: Mac Keith Press.)

Foley, J. (1983) 'The athetoid syndrome. A review of a personal series.' *Journal of Neurology, Neurosurgery and Psychiatry*, **46**, 289–298.

Howlin, P. (1998) *Children with Autism and Asperger Syndrome: a Guide for Practitioners and Carers.* Chichester: John Wiley.

Ingram, T.T.S. (1964) *Paediatric Aspects of Cerebral Palsy.* Edinburgh/London: E. & S. Livingstone.

Landau, W.M., Kleffner, F.R. (1957) 'Syndrome of acquired aphasia with convulsive disorder in children.' *Neurology*, **7**, 523–530.

Mantovani, J.F., Landau, W.M. (1980) 'Acquired aphasia with convulsive disorder: course and prognosis.' *Neurology*, **30**, 524–529.

Mesibov, G.B., Schopler, E., Hearsey, K.A. (1994) 'Structured teaching.' *In:* Schopler, E., Mesibov, G.B. (Eds.) *Behavioural Issues in Autism.* New York: Plenum Press, pp. 195–207.

Millar, D., Light, J., Schlosser, R. (2000) 'The impact of augmentative and alternative communication on natural speech development: a meta-analysis.' *Paper presented at the August 2000 Meeting of the International Society for Augmentative and Alternative Communication, Washington, DC.*

Mutter, V., Vargha-Khadem, F. (2000) 'Neuropsychology and educational management.' *In:* Neville, B., Goodman, R. (Eds.) *Congenital Hemiplegia. Clinics in Developmental Medicine No. 150.* London: Mac Keith Press, pp. 179–194.

Netsell, R. (1991) *A Neurobiologic View of Speech Production and the Dysarthrias.* San Diego: Singular Publishing.

Rowland, C., Schweigert, P. (2000) 'Tangible symbols, tangible outcomes.' *Augmentative and Alternative Communication*, **16**, 61–78.

Stanley, F., Blair, E., Alberman, E. (2000) *Cerebral Palsies: Epidemiology and Causal Pathways. Clinics in Developmental Medicine No. 151.* London: Mac Keith Press.

Thomas, A.P., Bax, M.C.O., Smyth, D.P.L. (1989) *The Health and Social Needs of Young Adults with Physical Disabilities. Clinics in Developmental Medicine No. 106.* London: Mac Keith Press.

Trevarthen, C., Aitken, K., Papoudi, D., Robarts, J. (1996) *Children with Autism: Diagnosis and Interventions to Meet Their Needs*. London: Jessica Kingsley.

Vance, M. (1991) 'Educational and therapeutic approaches used with a child presenting with acquired aphasia with convulsive disorder (Landau–Kleffner syndrome).' *Child Language Teaching and Therapy*, 7, 41–60.

4

ASSESSING CHILDREN FOR AUGMENTATIVE AND ALTERNATIVE COMMUNICATION

Helen Cockerill and Prue Fuller

Since the early 1980s the assessment of children requiring augmentative and alternative communication (AAC) has involved a team approach. Because it is essential to have an holistic understanding of the child, a range of professionals is usually involved in gathering information about a child's abilities and needs in order to make informed decisions about appropriate AAC systems, techniques and support. As in many other areas of clinical practice, specialist AAC teams have aspired to multidisciplinary, interdisciplinary and transdisciplinary team working over the past 20 years. A more collaborative approach is now being advocated, in which team members bring their unique expertise to the assessment process, but which places the child and family at the heart of the decision-making process (Beukelman and Mirenda 1998; Blackstone 1994, 1995b). Other chapters in this book describe the way in which AAC teams must work in collaboration with families and schools if AAC is to be implemented successfully. This chapter will focus on the contribution of specialist AAC professionals once assessment has been requested by a child's school, community team or family. Most children requiring AAC will already be known to local services and may be in receipt of a range of therapy and education services. In most countries AAC services are likely to be organized in two or three tiers. A minority of children with severe speech impairments will be receiving services from community clinics, with the majority receiving input from secondary level child development teams, preschool services, schools (special provision or mainstream) or mainstream support services. While some special school and child health services will include professionals with AAC knowledge, many children will require referral to specialist AAC teams.

AAC teams

The exact composition of the team involved in assessment is highly variable. There are no studies comparing the composition and practices of AAC teams across international boundaries, and few published reviews of the organization of services. However, descriptions of services within countries or states are often presented at international conferences such as those held by the International Society for Augmentative and Alternative Communication (ISAAC). Factors determining the composition of teams are often service-driven rather than based on best practice. In the UK, where many of the AAC teams are located within the tertiary level of the National Health Service, assessment team members have traditionally included speech and language therapists to advise on receptive language and capacity for natural speech; occupational and/or physiotherapists to advise on seating, positioning and motor control; and rehabilitation engineers to advise on the technical aspects of matching a child's abilities to the available technology. There may also be medical input from a paediatrician or paediatric neurologist, particularly when the AAC team is located within a more general childhood disability service (Jones *et al.* 1990). It is rare for teachers to be included in such teams. In the UK there are two national assessment centres, funded partly by the Department for Education and Employment, whose staff include teachers, speech and language therapists, occupational therapists, technicians and researchers. Some local education authorities have specialist AAC teachers who work collaboratively with speech and language therapists, occupational therapists and physiotherapists where possible. The weakness of this approach may be a focus on the use of technology for recording and accessing the curriculum, with a relatively lower priority being given to low-tech communication systems (signing, symbols, etc.) and the development of social skills.

In some countries where AAC is a newer concept, teams that cross the traditional health/education divide are emerging. For example, Poland has established a number of AAC centres where teachers and therapists are able to work together, and in the Indian Institute of Cerebral Palsy in Calcutta joint assessments by teachers and therapists are undertaken. In the USA special educators are likely to be core members of the team alongside speech and language pathologists and occupational therapists (Swengel and Marquette 1997). Psychologists may also be core members, and in Europe and Scandinavia have often taken a lead role in assessment and training.

The limitations of individual teams necessitate collaborative working with the child's community therapists and teachers. In some cases, particularly in the USA, schools or community teams may call in an individual AAC consultant, usually a professional from a speech and language pathology or special education background who has years of experience of implementing AAC programmes. The consultant will bring specialist knowledge to the assessment process and work collaboratively with the family and local team.

The assessment setting

Children may travel with their families and local team members to a centre for assessment. The advantages of this arrangement include the team having access to a range of assessment materials such as vision testing equipment, chairs and other positioning aids, a wide range of switches, communication devices, adapted toys, etc. Equipment is available for trial and adaptations can be quickly made. Families are able to view a range of AAC devices and materials. The disadvantages include possible fatigue for the child and family, apprehension at being in an unfamiliar environment, lack of involvement of some family and local team members, and possible inability to access the child's specialist equipment. As part of an holistic assessment the team will need to establish a realistic picture of how the child communicates within her/his everyday environment, and to build up an understanding of her/his communication needs. This may be difficult to achieve if the child is in an unfamiliar setting, therefore some teams choose to send core members to the child's home or school to carry out the assessment. One UK project (the ACE Centre Telenet Project, Oxford) is currently investigating a method of working with children and their local teams via regular video conferencing and data exchange. This allows direct access to the expertise of a specialist team without the disruption of a long journey or removing the child from her/his everyday environment.

In order to circumvent some of the limitations of traditional centre-based assessment, a range of assessment methods have been devised. These are described below.

Assessment methods

INTERVIEWS

As part of the information-gathering process, the parents and local professionals may be interviewed (either informally during the assessment, and/or on the telephone or through questionnaires) about the child's skills, communication opportunities and needs. The interview can also provide an opportunity to listen to the parents' views on the child's current communication, their understanding of the causes of their child's difficulties, and their expectations with regards to AAC, both positive and negative. There may be differences between parents and the local team, which will need to be addressed in the process of consensus-building and action planning.

A range of semi-structured interview tools is available to explore these areas with the child's communication partners. These include developmental checklists, *e.g.* the Receptive–Expressive Emergent Language Scale (Bzoch and League 1991) and the MacArthur Communicative Development Inventories (Fenson *et al.* 1993), or descriptive tools, *e.g.* the Pragmatics Profile (Dewart and Summers 1995). Although developmental checklists are not designed specifically for children with disabilities, they can obtain useful information about a child if used in conjunction with informal observation methods.

VIDEOS/OBSERVATION

Families and/or local team members may be asked to provide video tapes of the child communicating at home or school, in a range of communication situations. These can then be used as a basis for discussion within the assessment session. This can be particularly important when assessing children with esoteric or idiosyncratic communication signals. 'Dynamic assessment' involves joint analysis of the video by the family and the AAC team, which can highlight a child's strengths and difficulties and can lead on to suggestions of specific techniques to facilitate interaction (Kublin *et al.* 1998).

Several studies investigating typical interaction patterns between parents and non-speaking children have used a technique in which the parent is offered a set of materials and asked to interact with her/his child as if at home (Light *et al.* 1985a,b,c; McConachie and Ciccognani 1995; Pennington and McConachie 1999). Such techniques can provide valuable information about the range of communication modes and functions used by the child and so can be employed as part of the assessment process. The same studies have demonstrated that a wider range of functions are used by the child in semi-scripted elicitation procedures with skilled clinicians. It is therefore desirable that an AAC team develop procedures in which a range of functions can be elicited. These may include adapted games and play situations that will be fun for the child but provide structured observation opportunities for the team (Price 1995).

A range of procedures will be used during the assessment session(s) to build up a picture of the child's skills. Because of the heterogeneous nature of the population referred for consideration of AAC, there can be no standardized assessment. A range of AAC techniques and devices may be explored within the assessment in order to observe a child's responses. The specific activities will be determined by the child's level of experience, skill and needs. These may be anything from offering choices using objects, through directing games either in a low-tech format (symbol cards or charts) or using voice output communication aids (VOCAs), to trialing predictive typing software on the computer. However, there is general consensus that the following areas should be considered in assessment: (i) motor skills, (ii) hearing, (iii) vision and visual perception, (iv) cognitive abilities, (v) language comprehension, (vi) literacy, (vii) natural speech, (viii) general health.

Motor skills assessment
It is unlikely that a child will undergo a full motor examination as part of an AAC assessment. This type of 'maximal assessment' would be time-consuming and inappropriate, as information should be available from local sources. However, the AAC team will wish to establish how the child's current seating and physical management programme impact on access to communication. In children with motor impairments, positioning can have major effects on a range of functional skills (Pope *et al*. 1994, Myhr *et al*. 1995). The effects of positioning on a child's ability to see, to orientate towards communication partners, to use hands/head/feet to point or press switches/keyboards, and to use natural speech must be considered in the assessment process.

When considering the most appropriate method of accessing a symbol chart or voice output communication aid, or the child's ability to use manual signs, it is important to consider the child's abilities when tired and ill as well as when in good health. Communication should not be precluded when the child is functioning at less than optimal levels. Accessing should use the child's most reliable and efficient motor movements so that effort can be directed towards the content of communication rather than the motor act. This can be a potential source of disagreement between team members, some of whom may see technology as a tool to develop motor skills rather than for the prime purpose of communication. Similarly, the amount of physical support required for efficient communication may be different from that which encourages the development of motor skills. Such issues must be addressed in the AAC assessment to prevent confusion and conflict of interests. Parents will have their own set of priorities, and children should also be offered the chance to express an opinion as to their preferred options for positioning, the optimal degree of physical support and accessing.

An area of motor functioning that has received little research attention is the possible long-term effect of repetitive use of a motor action to access technological devices. This issue of repetitive strain injury (RSI) was raised by Blackstone (1995a), who listed factors that may place people with disabilities at risk of developing RSI. These included poor posture, poor fitness levels, high stress, and repetitive use of the same part of the body, *e.g.* turning the head to activate a switch. General principles, such as providing a resting place or support (*e.g.* a head rest), consideration of small movements for accessing since these are easier to control than large movements, the notion that a person will have most control over movements in the middle of her/his total range of movement, and providing sensory feedback using auditory, visual and tactile options were proposed. Cerebral palsy is a non-progressive but not unchanging disorder of posture and movement (Bax 1964). This definition highlights the importance of repeated assessment in order to monitor how changes in physical skills impact on access to communication, and also how communication access methods impact on physical well-being.

Assessment of hearing

Movement disorders can make the accurate assessment of hearing problematic. A sound-based communication system (auditory scanning) may be considered appropriate for a child with an additional visual impairment, therefore it is vital to establish adequate hearing levels. Children with autistic spectrum disorders may show selective responses to sound, with such a lack of attention to speech that a hearing loss is suspected. Children with such complex needs may require comprehensive testing in specialist centres as part of, or prior to, AAC assessment.

Assessment of vision

While all children with disabilities should have had an assessment of vision and hearing as part of a general paediatric examination, those for whom visually based methods of communication are being considered may require additional assessment (Jones *et al.* 1990). In order to access visual systems, a child needs to be able to see, scan, perceive and interpret two-dimensional information. Children with motor impairments are known to be at risk of additional visual impairments, including oculo-motor, perceptual, primary visual and cortical visual disorders (Pellegrino 1997). In offering advice on appropriate visual materials, on the size, number and colour of symbols, and on the size, positioning and layout of symbol displays, the AAC team may need access to specialist visual assessment. Standardized assessments that use a preferential looking paradigm (*e.g.* Keeler cards) may be of value, but it is also important to have a range of assessment materials that allow functional vision assessment, *e.g.* toys and symbols of varying sizes, black-and-white *vs.* colour symbols.

Cognitive assessment

In the early 1980s many assessment models assumed that children needed to demonstrate they had acquired certain prerequisite skills, such as an understanding of cause and effect, before being introduced to AAC. For example, Shane (1981) stated that a cognitive level of Piaget's sensorimotor stage 5 (mental age of at least 18 months) must be reached before AAC intervention took place. In part this begs the question of whether it is possible to establish a child's cognitive level with certainty, particularly if that child has severe physical impairment. Testing of cognitive skills in this population poses many problems, as children may not be able to access test materials. Some tests, such as the Leiter International Performance Scales (1952) can be adapted for eye-pointing but have not been standardized for those conditions. Also it might be argued that the examiner would be testing the expressive skill of eye-pointing as much as the child's cognitive ability. Some children do develop eye-pointing skills spontaneously, whereas other children may need to be taught to use such strategies. Children with eye-movement disorders may be disadvantaged by such assessment methods. Similarly, when assessing a young child with autism the test results may reflect difficulties with compliance rather than cognitive limitations.

In addition, the concept of what constitutes AAC intervention has perhaps changed over the past 20 years. AAC professionals now have access to a wide range of technology and techniques to enhance and promote communication whatever the child's cognitive level. Definitions of AAC are no longer confined to alternative forms of symbolic communication. Strategies such as aided language stimulation (Goossens *et al.* 1992), the TEACCH approach (Mesibov *et al.* 1994) in which spoken language is accompanied by visual cues, and the use of objects of reference (Park 1997) where a child is consistently offered a meaningful object immediately before or during an activity, may benefit children who are not able to demonstrate the cognitive skills of a typically developing 18-month-old. There are also many stories of the cognitive abilities of non-speaking individuals only becoming apparent after the introduction of AAC. For these and other reasons there has been a tendency to reject the notion of prerequisites for AAC intervention on the premise that AAC could circumvent even the most severe impairment (Blackstone 1994).

A complete disregard for the role of cognition in AAC would, however, be foolish. There is a danger of setting unrealistic targets and presenting children with over-complex systems if cognitive factors are not monitored through ongoing assessment. Recent research by Light and her colleagues at Pennsylvania State University (reported by Blackstone 1999b) investigates the learning demands of symbol-based electronic communication aids. When typically developing children between the ages of 2.5 and 5 years were given instruction in the use of such devices in play situations, the difficulties posed by the learning and use of graphic methods of communication were highlighted. It is hoped that such data will lead to a more reasoned consideration of the cognitive demands of particular AAC systems and techniques.

Language comprehension assessment
As with cognitive assessment, very few tests have been standardized for use with non-speaking children who rely on nonverbal communication. The Comprehension scale of the Reynell Developmental Language Scales – Revised (Reynell and Huntley 1985) was standardized for eye-pointing, but the latest version of the test requires physical manipulation of the test materials. Some receptive language sub-tests from other test batteries may be suitable for adaptation (without standardization). Adaptations might include cutting up test materials and spacing them to allow for eye-pointing, or listener-assisted scanning, *i.e.* the examiner points to each option in turn and waits for the child to indicate her/his choice. Tests that use multiple-choice pointing formats to assess aspects of comprehension include the Clinical Evaluation of Language Fundamentals – Preschool (Wigg *et al.* 1992), the Clinical

Evaluation of Language Fundamentals – Revised (Semel *et al.* 1987), and the Peabody Picture Vocabulary Test – Revised (Dunn and Dunn 1981). Attempts have been made to computerize tests with a multiple-choice format, but these presuppose that the child has excellent accessing skills in which a switch can be depressed when an on-screen cursor scans the options. Unfortunately, few young or severely disabled children have such reliable access competence.

For younger children, or those who do not appear to understand picture materials, developmental checklists such as the Receptive–Expressive Emergent Language Scale (Bzoch and League 1991) or the MacArthur Developmental Inventory (Fenson *et al.* 1993) can be used to get a feeling for the child's level of ability, although it should be remembered that these tools describe the development of the typical, non-disabled population.

A range of tools have been developed to describe the communication skills, including language or pre-linguistic understanding, of the multiply disabled population. The Pre-Verbal Communication Schedule (PVCS) (Kiernan and Reid 1987), the Early Communication Assessment (ECA) (Coupe O'Kane and Goldbart 1998) and Assessing Communication (Latham and Miles 1997) are typical examples. These tools are designed to record the observations of the child's familiar communication partners, to document the child's current levels of functioning within everyday environments, and to provide guidance for intervention. All adopt a developmental perspective but do not necessarily attach age levels to the skills described. The PVCS and ECA provide reliability data. While it would be impossible to complete these assessments during an AAC assessment, they can be used by local teams, and can provide a useful structure for asking families about their children's communication skills. Families and those who are in direct contact with the child can bring to the assessment situation their observations about a child's understanding. In the situation where a child's signals are difficult to interpret, the AAC team may need to ask careful questions of the familiar communication partners in order to specify what exactly the child does that tells them that s/he has understood. Familiar carers may also be unaware of the type of nonverbal supports to language comprehension they are using such as pointing, eye-gaze, showing objects, repetitive routines, etc. (von Tetzchner and Martinsen 2000).

The aim of assessing language comprehension is not to establish candidacy for AAC intervention but to estimate the size of the discrepancy between a child's language under-standing and expressive skills, and to provide at least initial guidance on appropriate implementation strategies.

Assessing literacy

In children with limited speech, AAC can provide a route into literacy, but literacy skills can also be part of a child's communication system. Children who are even partly literate may be able to access vocabulary on a low- or high-tech system through printed words, or may use initial letter cues, possibly in combination with symbols. Word and letter recognition can be assessed using finger/fist/eye-pointing, or selecting words from lists/grids on the computer if the child has effective accessing skills. Children who already have some experience of symbol systems may have learnt to recognize some of the printed words that have been paired with the symbols on their charts. Skills in reading the same words in a different context and novel words should be investigated. Children who can spell, at least phonetically, can use these skills to generate messages on dedicated or computer-based AAC devices.

Assessing natural speech

With the exception of children with a tracheostomy, most children referred for AAC assessment will have some degree of vocal ability. This may be anywhere from crying to indicate distress, to dysarthric speech.

There are few dysarthria assessments designed specifically for children, and the sort of maximal assessment procedure of tools such as the Paediatric Oral Skills Profile (Brindley *et al.* 1996) are inappropriate for the AAC assessment setting. Sections of The Apraxia Profile (Hickman 1997), while not aimed at the dysarthric population, can be used as a screen of involuntary and voluntary oral skills, single sound production, and word and phrase repetition. However, a measure of oral motor skills is not the same as assessing a child's 'comprehensibility', *i.e.* how well s/he can be understood by her/his communication partners. The child's ability to use natural speech effectively may depend as much on a communication partner's ability to understand as on the extent of the dysarthria. Parents and those in everyday contact with a child are likely to understand more than the AAC team, as they are able to recruit a large store of personal information about the speaker.

Speech production can be influenced by a range of factors including postural stability, stress/excitement, fatigue, epilepsy, hearing and general health, and therefore can be highly variable within one individual. Comprehensibility is a concept that also takes into account the listener's skills. Attempts have been made to quantify intelligibility/comprehensibility, both for the purpose of measuring treatment efficacy and to assist in decision-making. For example, the Children's Speech Intelligibility Measure (Wilcox and Morris 1997) and the Index of Augmented Speech Comprehension in Children (Dowden 1997) both involve recording children's speech and then measuring a listener's ability to identify the words, from a restricted list. Again, such procedures are unlikely to be practical within AAC assessment but could be useful research or outcome measures when investigating the effects of articulation work or AAC intervention. Within the framework of a pragmatic and holistic AAC assessment it is probable that judgements of the degree to which natural speech will meet the child's communication need will be subjective.

In the majority of AAC assessments the issue of how AAC might impact on natural speech development will be raised. Many parents and professionals fear that focusing on AAC will hinder the development of speech, either because the child will depend on the AAC system or because resources will be directed away from articulation therapy towards AAC. Few data are available either on the natural course of dysarthria or, more specifically, on the efficacy of treatment (Coombes 1984). Speech involves the highest level of sensorimotor integration, postural control, breath and phonatory coordination, and highly differentiated selective movements of the palate, lips and tongue. For this reason many speech and language therapists are highly sceptical about the value of traditional speech therapy with the severely disabled population. In the historical candidacy model of AAC, teams were required to decide which children should receive articulation work and which should receive

AAC intervention (*e.g.* Shane and Bashir 1980). Such simplistic 'either/or' decisions are no longer appropriate.

Many children will continue to use speech, even of very low intelligibility, as their preferred method of communication with familiar partners. This should not be dismissed even if unintelligible to the AAC team. There is a growing interest in the use of voice recognition software for those with dysarthric speech as well as for unimpaired speakers, an area that may have considerable potential to support speakers of low intelligibility (Donegan 2000). More traditional supplementation strategies such as initial letter cues or pointing to symbols to indicate a change of topic can significantly increase intelligibility (see Yorkston *et al.* 1999) and may help in reconciling parents to a child's need for AAC with less skilled listeners.

There are no published research studies that have been designed specifically to monitor the effects of AAC intervention on natural speech. A recent meta-analysis of AAC intervention studies by Miller *et al.* (2000) provided some evidence that speech production increases or remains unchanged. Conclusions are tentative due to the limitations of the original studies. Relatively small numbers of AAC intervention studies could be included as most did not document changes in speech production, and many contained significant methodological flaws. The 50 studies in the analysis included individuals with autism or learning disability of varying severity, and most involved sign language rather than graphic symbols or technology. Anecdotal evidence, however, would indicate that the use of AAC encourages rather than discourages the use of natural speech.

General health assessment
Communication for children with physical disabilities can be effortful, both physically and cognitively. The child's general state of health can have dramatic effects on posture and physical function, attention and learning. Epilepsy and the medication to control the condition can produce variability in functional skills and a child's nutritional status can impact on comfort, energy and attention levels. Children with disordered oromotor skills may have severe dysphagia, which in turn can compromise respiratory health if aspiration is present. While eating and drinking are unlikely to be the main focus of an AAC assessment, a child who is failing to thrive or experiencing frequent chest infections, and who may be missing schooling due to hospitalizations or physiotherapy sessions, is not in a position to benefit fully from intervention directed at communication. For this reason the AAC team will need to gather information in these areas and discuss the importance of such issues with those caring for the child (Cass *et al.* 1999).

Profiling a child's abilities
The AAC team is aiming to build a picture of each child's specific capabilities in the areas outlined above, in order to make appropriate recommendations. In 1989 Light proposed a model of communicative competence that has been used by AAC professionals when describing children's unique abilities. Another influential model in the field of AAC has been the Participation Model developed by Beukelman and Mirenda (1998), which lays equal stress on the child's communicative environment. Figure 4.1 represents a synthesis

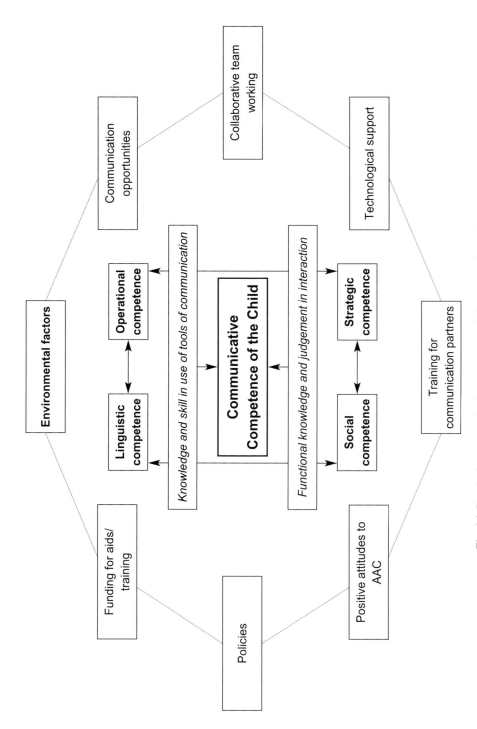

Fig. 4.1. Developing communicative competence within a supportive environment.

of these models. In making recommendations the AAC assessment team will be attempting to consider all aspects of this model.

Communicative competence is defined as "the quality or state of being *functionally adequate* in daily communication, or of having *sufficient knowledge, judgement, and skill* to communicate" (Light 1989). A child's capabilities can be described in terms of four interrelated areas:

- *Linguistic competence*—mastery of the native language of the home and community, and the linguistic code of the AAC system, *e.g.* manual signs, pictures, symbols, printed words.
- *Operational competence*—technical skills to operate the system of communication, *e.g.* accuracy and speed in eye-pointing, switch operation, joystick operation, etc., including sensory, perceptual and cognitive skills.
- *Social competence*—context-dependent interaction skills, *e.g.* initiating, maintaining and terminating interaction, turn-taking, confidence, motivation, using a range of communication functions, etc.
- *Strategic competence*—flexibility in communicating, *e.g.* use of a variety of modes of communication, repair strategies, providing clarification, etc.

Consideration of the child's skills in these areas can highlight intervention priorities. For example a young physically disabled child who has age-appropriate language understanding and uses a range of nonverbal strategies to initiate and maintain interaction but who has little intelligible speech will require the introduction of a symbol-based expressive language system (low- and high-tech), with consideration of the most appropriate accessing methods. Intervention for a young autistic child with impaired social interaction skills and limited language understanding may focus on the introduction of a symbol-based system to facilitate comprehension, with strategies to increase compliance and turn-taking.

Assessing the communication environment

The outer circle of Figure 4.1 includes factors that are considered important to support a child in developing communicative competence. An holistic assessment must incorporate consideration of the environment in order to identify possible opportunity barriers (Beukelman and Mirenda 1998) and put in place measures to minimize these barriers. Many of these areas are covered by other authors in this volume, therefore only a brief listing of environmental factors will be given here.

COMMUNICATION OPPORTUNITIES

To develop competence in using an AAC system a child needs opportunities for functional and meaningful communication in a range of daily activities. Research studies continue to report that AAC systems are often only used in specific speech and language therapy sessions. Anticipation of needs and an overprotective attitude from carers can reduce the chances of failure, but also the opportunities to develop skills. Children may have a limited number of partners and have established patterns of communication with those partners in which it may be difficult to incorporate AAC strategies. Negotiation between AAC professionals and carers may be required to identify realistic and appropriate opportunities for decision-making and independence.

COLLABORATIVE TEAM WORKING

The recommendations from the AAC assessment should not be a list of actions for the child's family and local team to put into practise. Goals of intervention should arise from collaborative problem-solving and include clear lines of responsibility for specific tasks such as seeking funding, producing symbol charts, adapting supportive seating, etc.

TECHNOLOGICAL SUPPORT

Electronic equipment requires maintenance, wheelchair mounting systems may need to be set up, communication software packages are likely to need customizing, and low-tech symbol systems need to be produced and maintained. The technological support for any AAC system must be identified, again with clear allocation of responsibility if systems are to be available and accessible to the child.

TRAINING FOR COMMUNICATION PARTNERS

Those in close contact with a child may have training needs in a variety of areas. Operating unfamiliar electronic devices is an obvious target, but perhaps more important is the area of interaction. Training can produce significant improvements in the quality of adults' facilitation of children's communication (McConachie and Pennington 1997). Responsibility for training may devolve to local teams or come from follow-up visits from the assessment team.

Adult AAC users have identified qualities that are desirable in communication partners (Blackstone 1999a). These included having real conversations, empathy, a genuine interest in what is being communicated, an ease in communicating with an AAC user, an ability to understand natural speech, and patience when an AAC device is being used. Undesirable characteristics included finishing sentences, doing something else while the user is formulating a message, and insisting on the use of the AAC system when messages can be conveyed by other means. When considering the needs of children it may be necessary to add the importance of modelling the use of the AAC system. Children will be largely dependent on their adult communication partners to provide appropriate vocabulary and demonstrate its use.

POSITIVE ATTITUDES TO AAC

AAC may be perceived as having lower status than natural speech (Woll and Barnett 1998). Self-esteem and feelings of worth in relation to an AAC system are likely to be important factors in motivating children to use a system, particularly in the absence of role-models, and could easily be undermined through negative comments from communication partners. Adults using a child's AAC system in conjunction with speech may help to raise its status as well as providing a model of use.

POLICIES

Policies at governmental, local authority and school level can have a profound impact on the individual child. Integration/inclusion policies can be beneficial or detrimental depending on the adequacy of support for AAC in a particular environment. Policies on provision of therapy services to children in different diagnostic groups can lead to discrepancies in levels of provision. Policies that specify that electronic communication aids can be used only in school, and not at home, can impede learning. Policy-making may not be directly within the control of the AAC team, but the ramifications for the individual child must be considered.

FUNDING

Computer-based systems, dedicated communication aids and low-tech AAC systems will all have funding implications. These will include not just the purchase and maintenance of equipment, but also training for families and local professionals, and therapy and teaching resources. The funding of AAC equipment and intervention services is a complex process within and across countries. In certain countries children have a legal right to assistive technology. In the USA for example, the Technology-Related Assistance for Individuals with Disabilities Act, Amendments of (1994) and the use of Individual Education Plans mandates that assistive technology be considered for children, and school districts must provide that equipment. However, the mandate is not funded, so that if the budget is exhausted, equipment will not be funded. In Canada, all citizens have the right to free health care under the Canada Health Act (1984), but the interpretation as to what constitutes health care varies. In Ontario it includes assistive devices, whereas in other provinces such as Alberta and British Colombia it does not. Similarly in the UK, if a child has a Statement of Special Educational Need that clearly specifies the need for AAC systems and their support, the Local Education Authority should fund provision. In reality few statements are sufficiently specific. Many children rely on charitable funds for the purchase of equipment, but funding rarely includes support. The process of application for funds can be a time-consuming and lengthy task, with many children experiencing a wait of months or even years. AAC assessment centres may have a loan bank of equipment, which can allow a child to trial a particular device to ensure it is the most appropriate option, and possibly demonstrate the effectiveness of the recommendations to funding authorities. Recommendations arising from assessment should include a funding plan that gives at least an initial estimate of the amount of funding required, and specifies who will have responsibility for pursuing that funding.

Summary

The assessment of children for AAC is a complex process, which requires a collaborative team approach. The child, the family, local professionals and the specialist AAC team will all contribute to a process that seeks to review the child's current skills, establish communication needs and consider the potential of a range of AAC systems, technology and techniques to meet those needs. It will be necessary to identify the resources available to support AAC intervention, and to establish the need for equipment, training and opportunities for communication, in addition to choosing an appropriate AAC system.

The majority of children will require regular reassessment. The responsibility of monitoring the performance of the child, and environment, in meeting the goals arising from the assessment may be devolved to the local team. As a child's communication skills and needs change, reassessment with a specialist team may be required, particularly if progression to a more powerful electronic device is being considered. The AAC team may also be involved in delivering training and some degree of ongoing support to the child's family or school. Recommendations as to the frequency, location and nature of the review process will depend on the child's rate of learning, the level of expertise in the child's community and funding.

REFERENCES

Bax, M.C.O. (1964) 'Terminology and classification of cerebral palsy.' *Developmental Medicine and Child Neurology*, **6**, 296–297.

Beukelman, D.R., Mirenda, P. (1998) *Augmentative and Alternative Communication: Management of Severe Communication Disorders in Children and Adults*. Baltimore: Paul H. Brookes.

Blackstone, S. (1994) 'What master clinicians do and think.' *Augmentative Communication News*, **7** (1), 5.

—— (1995a) 'Repetitive strain injury and AAC.' *Augmentative Communication News*, **8** (2), 1–4.

—— (1995b) '2,4,6,8, How do we collaborate?' *Augmentative Communication News*, **8** (4), 1–3.

—— (1999a) 'Communication partners: E-mail survey.' *Augmentative and Alternative Communication*, **12** (1/2), 6–7.

—— (1999b) 'Improving AAC technologies for young children.' *Augmentative Communication News*, **12** (6), 6–7.

Brindley, C., Cave, D., Crane, S., Moffat, V. (1996) *Paediatric Oral Skills Package*. London: Whurr.

Bzoch, K.R., League, R. (1991) *The Receptive and Expressive Emergent Language Scale, 2nd Edn*. Baltimore: University Park Press.

Cass, H., Price, K., Reilly, S., Wisbeach, A., McConachie, H. (1999) 'A model for the assessment and management of children with multiple disabilities.' *Child: Care, Health and Development*, **25**, 191–211.

Coombes, K. (1984) 'Speech therapy.' In: Yule, W., Rutter, M. (Eds.) *Language Development and Disorders. Clinics in Developmental Medicine No. 101/102*. London: Mac Keith Press, pp. 350–366.

Coupe O'Kane, J., Goldbart, J. (1998) *Communication Before Speech*. London: David Fulton.

Dewart, H., Summers, S. (1995) *The Pragmatics Profile of Everyday Communication in Pre-school and School-aged Children*. Windsor: NFER-Nelson.

Donegan, M. (2000) *Voice Recognition Technology in Education: Factors for Success*. Oxford: ACE Centre.

Dowden, P. (1997) 'Augmentative and alternative communication decision making for children with severely unintelligible speech.' *Augmentative and Alternative Communication*, **13**, 48–58.

Dunn, L.M., Dunn, L.M. (1981) *Peabody Picture Vocabulary Test – Revised*. Circle Pines, MN: American Guidance Service.

Fenson, L., Dale, P.S., Reznick, J.S., Thal, D., Hartung, J.P., Pethick, S., Reilly, J.S. (1993) *MacArthur Communicative Development Inventories*. California: Singular.

Goosens, C., Crain, S., Elder, P. (1992) *Engineering the Preschool Environment for Interactive Symbolic Communication*. Birmingham, AL: Southeast Augmentative Communication Conference Publications.

Hickman, L.A. (1997) *The Apraxia Profile*. San Antonio, TX: Psychological Corporation.

Jones, S. Jolleff, N., McConachie, H., Wisbeach, A. (1990) 'A model for assessment of children for augmnetative communication systems.' *Child Language, Teaching and Therapy*, **6**, 305–321.

Kiernan, C., Reid, B. (1987) *Pre-verbal Communication Schedule*. Windsor: NFER-Nelson.

Kublin, K.S., Wetherby, A.M., Crais, E.R., Prizant, B.M. (1998) 'Using dynamic assessment within collaborative contexts.' *In:* Wetherby, A., Warren, S., Reichle, J. (Eds.) *Transitions in Prelinguistic Communication*. Baltimore: Paul H. Brookes, pp. 285–312.

Latham, C., Miles, A. (1997) *Assessing Communication*. London: David Fulton.

Leiter, R.G. (1952) *Leiter International Performance Scale*. Wood Vale, IL: Stoelting.

Light, J. (1989) 'Toward a definition of communicative competence for individuals using augmentative and alternative communication systems.' *Augmentative and Alternative Communication*, **5**, 137–144.

—— Collier, B., Parnes, P. (1985a) 'Communicative interaction between nonspeaking physically disabled children and their primary caregivers: Part I. Discourse patterns.' *Augmentative and Alternative Communication*, **1**, 74–83.

—— —— —— (1985b) 'Communicative interaction between nonspeaking physically disabled children and their primary caregivers: Part II. Communicative function.' *Augmentative and Alternative Communication*, **1**, 98–107.

—— —— —— (1985c) 'Communicative interaction between nonspeaking physically disabled children and their primary caregivers: Part III. Modes of communication.' *Augmentative and Alternative Communication*, **1**, 125–133.

McConachie, H., Ciccognani, A. (1995) 'What's in the box? Assessing physically disabled children's communication skills.' *Journal of Child Language, Teaching and Therapy*, **11**, 253–262.

—— Pennington, L. (1997) 'In-service training for schools on augmentative and alternative communication.' *European Journal of Disorders of Communication*, **32**, 277–288.

Mesibov, G.B., Schopler, E., Hearsey, K. (1994) 'Structured teaching.' *In:* Schopler, E., Mesibov, G. (Eds.) *Behavioural Issues in Autism.* New York: Plenum Press, pp. 195–207.

Miller, D., Light, J., Schlosser, R. (2000) 'The impact of AAC on natural speech development: a meta-analysis.' *Paper presented at the 9th Biennial Conference of the International Society for Augmentative and Alternative Communication, Washington, DC, August 2000.*

Myhr, U., von Wendt, L., Norrlin, S., Radell, U. (1995) 'Five-year follow-up of functional sitting position in children with cerebral palsy.' *Developmental Medicine and Child Neurology*, **37**, 587–596.

Park, K. (1997) 'How do objects become objects of reference? A review of the literature on objects of reference and a proposed model for the use of objects in communication.' *British Journal of Special Education*, **24**, 108–113.

Pellegrino, L. (1997) 'Cerebral palsy.' *In:* Batshaw, M. (Ed.) *Children with Disabilities, 4th Edn.* Baltimore: Paul H. Brookes, pp. 499–528.

Pennington, L., McConachie, H. (1999) 'Mother–child interaction revisited: Communication with non-speaking physically disabled children.' *International Journal of Language and Communication Disorders*, **34**, 391–416.

Pope, P.M., Bowes, C.E., Booth, E. (1994) 'Postural control in sitting. The SAM system: evaluation of use over three years.' *Developmental Medicine and Child Neurology*, **36**, 241–252.

Price, K. (1995) 'Promoting successful communication: games and activities to encourage specific communication functions.' *Communication Matters*, **9** (2), 22–23.

Reynell, J., Huntley, M. (1985) *Reynell Developmental Language Scales – Revised. 2nd Edn.* Windsor: NFER-Nelson.

Semel, E., Wigg, E.H., Secord, W. (1997) *Clinical Evaluation of Language Fundamentals – Revised.* New York: Psychological Corporation.

Shane, H. (1981) 'Decision making in early augmentative communication system use.' *In:* Schiefelbusch, R., Bricker, D. (Eds.) Early Language: Acquisition and Intervention. Baltimore: University Park Press, pp. 389–425.

—— Bashir, A.S. (1980) 'Election criteria for the adoption of an augmentative communication system.' *Journal of Speech and Hearing Disorders*, **45**, 408–414

Swengel, K.E., Marquette, J.S. (1997) 'Service delivery in AAC.' *In:* Glennen, S.L., DeCoste, D.C. (Eds.) *Handbook of Augmentative and Alternative Communication.* San Diego: Singular, pp. 21–58.

von Tetzchner, S., Martinsen, H. (2000) *Introduction to Augmentative and Alternative Communication, 2nd Edn.* London: Whurr.

Wigg, E.H., Secord, W., Semel, E. (1992) *Clinical Evaluation of Language Fundamentals – Preschool.* New York: Psychological Corporation.

Wilcox, K., Morris, S. (1997) *Children's Speech Intelligibility Measure.* San Antonio: Psychological Corporation.

Woll, B., Barnett, S. (1998) 'Toward a sociolinguistic perspective on augmentative and alternative communication.' *Augmentative and Alternative Communication*, **14**, 200–211.

Yorkston, K.M., Beukelman, D.R., Strand, E.A., Bell, K.R. (1999) *Management of Motor Speech Disorders in Children and Adults, 2nd Edn.* Austin, TX: Pro-ed.

5
WORKING WITH FAMILIES TO INTRODUCE AUGMENTATIVE AND ALTERNATIVE COMMUNICATION SYSTEMS

Mats Granlund, Eva Björck-Åkesson, Cecilia Olsson and Bitte Rydeman

The function of communication intervention in the family system

For many years the importance of the family and the home environment for the development of language in children with disabilities has been stressed. Recently the family has been discussed also in relation to other roles and missions (Gallagher 1990, Björck-Åkesson *et al.* 2000). These new perspectives are based on the assumption that the family can be seen as a system, in which the child with disabilities is one of the members. The way the child affects the family is as important as the way the family affects the child, that is, the focus has been moved from language to communication and interaction. The family is regarded as an open system in constant interaction with surrounding systems. It is an entity with communicative needs in its own right and also a forum for communication intervention decisions. This development necessitates a discussion about the different roles and missions assigned to the family, different models for service delivery, and possible outcomes of communication intervention.

In Table 5.1 different focuses, desired outcomes, and methods of communication intervention are displayed and related to the roles and tasks of parents and professionals in intervention.

FAMILY AS DECISION MAKERS

Communication intervention services must stress the active participation of the family in the decision making. By this means the family and the child with disabilities can experience a sense of forming their own life (life projects, lifestyle, etc.) and a sense of continuity in the services obtained. If professionals take the role as experts who decide the goals and methods of intervention, the services obtained by the child with disabilities and her/his family tend to be fragmented and without a common aim (Granlund *et al.* 1998). Therefore the family must be given opportunities to be involved in decisions regarding assessment, goals and methods for communication intervention. This requires professionals to provide services based on collaborative problem-solving methods (Björck-Åkesson *et al.* 1996) and to use assessment material that facilitates parental participation.

TABLE 5.1
Roles and missions of the family in communication intervention

Focus	Goal/objective	Professional role in intervention	Role assigned to family	Family task
Family as decision makers	Family is actively involved in and perceives control over the communication intervention process	• Provide opportunities for involvement and control • Teach problem-solving strategies	• Decision maker • Service coordinator	• Express needs • Design goals and methods • Select from service options • Evaluate
The family as communicative environment	The child with disabilities interacts optimally with persons within the proximal environment and has a 'rich environment'	• Supervision and interaction coaching • Parents are given advice, adapted toys, etc. • Stimulation outside home is provided, *e.g.* day-care	• Providers of 'rich environment' • Interaction partners • Providing and maintaining assistive technology	• Stimulate child • Adapt environment to needs of child with disabilities
Family as consumers	Decrease in perceived family needs	• Assess needs • Fulfill needs	• Recipient of services	• Identify needs and problems • Use available services
Family in crisis	Family has a normal family life cycle and 'accepts' actual child, *e.g.* copes with grief reactions	• Crisis therapy • Respite care • Redefine behaviour of child with disabilities	• Patient • Client	• 'Solve/cope with emotional reactions' • Interpret and interact with child in a realistic fashion
Family as trainers	Optimal child development within specific area	• Teach training programme • Supervise parents	• Student • Trainer	• Implement programme designed by professionals

FAMILY AS COMMUNICATIVE ENVIRONMENT

The creation of a meaningful and sustainable environment is an important task in most families. Families organize and shape their members' activities, function and development through daily routines. In creating and maintaining routines, families respond to sometimes conflicting circumstances. This process has been called family accommodation (Gallimore *et al.* 1993, Leskinen 1994). The everyday routine does not exist in a social vacuum. It is shaped by surrounding ecocultural features such as: family subsistence and financial base; accessibility to educational services and health services; home security and convenience; domestic task and chore workload of the family; care tasks related to family members; social leisure activities; marital role relationships; social support; sources of information; and goals (Gallimore *et al.* 1996). Accommodation is a process common to all families. What accommodations are made depends on many factors including ecological constraints and resources, cultural beliefs and customs. Intervention can have two focuses in relation to the communicative environment. It can be aimed at the construction and maintenance of a daily routine containing interactions through which the child develops and functions optimally (Granlund and Olsson 1999); such interventions tend to be of low intensity and long term, they must be sensitive to other types of adjustments made by the family and accommodate to the changing needs of the family and the child with disabilities over time. The other focus is on integrating specific interventions and/or assistive technology into the family environment. Interventions that are not implemented or sustained are probably not well fitted to the existing daily routine and the many adaptations a family is already making. An example is the abandonment of AAC technical equipment for reasons such as: use of equipment complicates daily routines; use of equipment disrupts social relationships; maintenance of equipment adds routines (Parette and Brotherson 1996); equipment is not adapted to the family environment, *e.g.* symbols are not chosen together with the family (Björck-Åkesson 1993).

FAMILY AS CONSUMERS

In adapting to their circumstances, families tend to express needs, *i.e.* to come up with possible solutions to the problems they are experiencing (Bailey and Simeonsson 1988, Roll-Pettersson *et al.* 1999). Professionals must be careful not to make the family dependent upon them for solutions. If families become dependent they tend to develop a role as passive recipients of services (Dunst *et al.* 1994). They also tend to implement interventions only as they have been told to and without flexibility and generalization to new settings and/or skills. To avoid dependency four characteristics of need identification must be taken into consideration (Dunst *et al.* 1994): (1) there must be a concern in the family that something is not as it ought to be; (2) the family must make a judgement that the discrepancy is currently or will influence the family's or the child's function; (3) there must be an awareness in the family that there is a resource that will reduce the discrepancy between what is and what ought to be; and (4) there must be a recognition that there is a way of procuring a resource to meet the need. Families tend to ask for solutions that they have knowledge about (*e.g.* speech therapy) rather than describing the problem that they are experiencing, and professionals have a tendency to identify the desired solutions as the problem (*e.g.* not enough speech therapy) rather than seeing them as the solution. Therefore there can be misunderstandings so that the solution provided (the one asked for) does not match the problem the solution is intended to solve. Professionals as well as families must be skilled at defining the problem by reasoning backwards from asking for a solution to expressing the problem in terms of the difference between how it is and how it ought to be (Granlund and Olsson 1998).

FAMILY IN CRISIS

The birth of a child with disabilities is an affliction to the members of the family and a grieving process is started. This grieving process is probably lifelong, and different families and individuals within families tend to cope with the process in more or less competent ways. The degree of 'crisis' experienced by the family tends to vary over time, dependent on personality and life-history of individual family members, life-circumstances and critical events (Bailey and Simeonsson 1988, Lagerheim 1988, Roll-Pettersson 1997). It is probable that family members experience a more severe crisis immediately after the detection/onset of the child's disability (*e.g.* birth or accident causing impairment and disability), after diagnosis, and in conjunction with normal life events such as starting school. Over time though, the family and the individual family members develop coping mechanisms that help them when crisis is experienced. Interventions with a crisis focus are aimed at helping family members through 'crisis periods'. Another aim is to help family members to develop strategies for coping with recurring crisis-periods. The interventions are time-limited and in the form of crisis therapy focused on the emotional reactions of parents, respite care and interventions aimed at redefining the family members' perceptions of the child with disabilities. Communication intervention with this focus is aimed at redefining (*i.e.* explaining and interpreting differently) the behaviour of the child with disabilities and thereby also changing the way that family members respond to and interact with the child. Thus the active participation of parents in defining interactional problems and in assessing the communicative skills and resources of the child is important. Communication interventions aimed at redefining family members' perceptions of the child with disabilities must be implemented with caution since they build on the assumption that the family members need to change their perceptions of the child with disabilities. Thus, the professional is assigned an expert role. Research has shown that redefining interventions focused on child–parent interaction have positive effects only when the parents have stated a need for help with interacting with their child. Interaction interventions implemented without parental consent tend to have negative effects on parent–child interaction (Affleck *et al.* 1989, McCollum and Hemmeter 1997).

FAMILY AS TRAINERS

Historically, family involvement in the assessment and intervention process has evolved from intervention programmes in which parents implemented training methods designed by professionals. The rationale was twofold, first to save money and clinician time, second to insure frequent use of the trained skill in a natural environment. When family members are assigned to the role of trainer, the professional's task is to teach training rationale and training skills to the family member who then applies the learned skills in training the child with disabilities. Two types of trainer role can be identified: implementing a complete training programme and training of a limited set of specific skills. In implementing a complete training programme the parents must adhere to a set of training methods for which the outcome is predetermined. Such programmes are in many instances based on a developmental perspective, *i.e.* the family environment is used to train a set of skills in a predetermined 'developmental sequence'. The professional is seen as an expert who defines the goals and methods for intervention. Thus, it often requires considerable adaptation of family routines and parental/spouse commitment for extended time periods. In communication intervention, the outcome of such 'training programmes' seems to be positive on the child's language development; the effects on the child's interaction skills and actual interaction patterns is not well documented (McCollum and Hemmeter 1997). The effects of commitment to a training programme on family functioning has been reported as both positive and negative (Ketelaar *et al.* 1998). Probably, comprehensive training programmes suit families who anyhow would have prioritized structured parent–child activities as an important parental task. Using parents as trainers of a limited set of skills is based on short-term interventions that might just as well be focused on a functional perspective as on a developmental one. The professional might be seen as an expert but can also be perceived as a collaborator who defines goals and methods in collaboration with the family, based on problems perceived by the family members.

In summary, the focus for communication intervention may vary both within the services given to a certain family and child over time and between families and children. The focus chosen for intervention has consequences for both the desired outcomes of intervention and the roles assigned to the family. Accordingly, the impact of communication intervention on the family system will vary dependent on the focus for intervention.

AAC and the family system
INTRODUCING AAC WITHIN THE HOME: GETTING STARTED
Basic to communicative interaction is that development is transactional. Sameroff and Fiese (1990) state that developmental outcomes are the "product of the continuous dynamic interactions of the child and the experience provided by his or her family and social context". In early interaction between the parents and the child mutual adaptation processes are started. Barnard and Kelly (1990) describe four characteristics in the adaptation process, or what they call the "mutual adaptive dance". First, each of the participants in interaction must have a sufficient repertoire of behaviours, *i.e.* to see, to hear, to pay attention, to smile, body-adaptation, and predictability of responses; second, responses must be contingent; third, there needs to be a richness of interactive content; and fourth, the pattern of interaction must change over time. When a child has a severe disability with few possibilities for self-expression, there is a risk of ongoing disturbance to adaptation processes from an early stage. The rhythm of the mutual adaptive dance becomes asynchronous, and communication becomes difficult for both the child and the parents (Brodin 1991, Björck-Åkesson 1993, Light 1997a). With respect to the mutuality of the development of interaction and communication it is necessary to start intervention within the family in everyday life. To ensure

predictability and contingency of responses, richness of communicative interaction and a change of pattern over time, the close interaction in everyday life is the most effective situation for interventions that improve the mutual adaptive dance.

Research has shown that in interaction between children with severe communication disability and parents, the parents and child seem to form inverted images of each other (Björck-Åkesson 1993, Light 1997a). For example, parents tend to take more turns compared to children, children frequently miss turn opportunities, and parents take the lead in interactions by using a large number of initiatives, while the children follow the lead and take few initiatives. Children's communicative turns are usually responsive, either confirmations or denials. This makes it difficult to maintain the interaction over a series of communicative turns. However, parents often guide the child through a communicative turn and give support to the child in the interaction. The patterns of communicative interaction between young physically disabled children with speech impairment and their parents tend to be asymmetric. The parents control the interaction by occupying more of the interactional space, initiating more topics for conversation and exerting a high degree of summoning power in their turns. Thus research shows that the parent plays an important role in the development of communicative interaction. To ensure positive outcomes, intervention should be carried through in natural situations in everyday life and involve both the child and the parent/ facilitator. When the social environment is actively involved in the intervention process, changes will occur in both the child and other persons in the close environment.

An adaptation perspective implies that the child should be given possibilities to function better, based on already acquired ability (Granlund *et al.* 1995). The goal of intervention is then to increase the frequency of communicative functions already acquired and to introduce more complex functions gradually. Intervention based on an adaptation/compensation perspective is closely related to an ongoing assessment process focused on the possibilities for the child to develop communication that functions in everyday life with the family and other close persons. This implies that both the child's and the parent's communication need to be assessed and to be part of the intervention, and that collaboration between parents and professionals is necessary.

To start a process where the interaction between parents and children is used as a basis for the intervention process, video recordings from everyday life can be used to observe the parents' and children's communicative interaction. These recordings can be done by the parents or by professionals before each meeting. With the help of structured rating scales and observations parents can observe and analyse both their own and the child's contributions in the communicative interaction. Parents learn about the children's communicative competency by observing their turn-taking in the interaction and looking at the form, function and content of the children's communication. The parents also learn to observe their own strategies in the communicative interaction, *e.g.* following the child's lead, soliciting a shared focus, providing opportunities for interaction, expecting, pacing, modelling, providing appropriate language input, prompting, rewarding communicative attempts and structuring the environment (Light *et al.* 1986, Björck-Åkesson *et al.* 1997). Collaborative problem-solving strategies, where parents and professionals learn from each other, are the basis in the intervention process (Björck-Åkesson *et al.* 1996). Based on the video observations, descriptions and explanations of problems in the communicative interaction are formulated by the parents together with professionals. The parents are seen as experts on their everyday life and their own lifestyle and goals, and also on their child's everyday behaviour and the problems they experience. Professionals are experts on explanations related to diagnosis and their specific area of specialization. An important part of the problem solving is prioritizing problems for intervention. Goals are then based on problem descriptions, and intervention methods are deduced from problem explanations. The outcome of the interventions can be documented by goal attainment scaling (Kiresuk *et al.* 1994); the intervention plan needs to be revised every second to third month to ensure that the intervention adapts to changes over time.

In an intervention study with young children with physical disabilities, the model described above was used (Björck-Åkesson *et al.* 1997). It revealed that both children and parents developed their communicative competence in the dyadic interactions. In interviews during and after the intervention, parents commented that they learned to 'see' their child's competencies through the video observations and the discussions with the professionals. Parents also said that they learned about their own role in the child's development of communication, and could see how changes in their own communication affected the child's communication and vice versa. The parents reported that they had changed their attitudes to the role of professionals in the intervention process, from being expert-oriented to where professionals were seen not just as experts on child development and disability, but also as partners in the problem-solving process and as consultants. A conclusion was that the parents experienced that a common frame of reference in building communicative competence was established through the collaborative problem-solving process and enabled the parents to take an active part in the intervention process. Fundamental to collaboration in the intervention process is the expectancy that each family has of the professionals and the service-providing process. It seems that expectations need to be clearly articulated before intervention is started and also to be discussed during this process.

To sum up, the success of communicative interaction depends on the partners participating in the mutual adaptive dance. In communicative intervention with children both the parents and the children are main actors in the process. Simultaneously with learning the basics of communicative interaction—such as turn-taking, joint attention, initiating and maintaining interaction—AAC systems (*e.g.* manual signs, aided communication) can be introduced.

INCORPORATING MANUAL SIGNING INTO SPEECH-BASED COMMUNICATION

Manual signs are the most used form of AAC with hearing, intellectually disabled children (von Tetzchner and Hygum Jensen 1996). Some of the reasons could be that there is no demand on the child for prerequisite language skills (Kangas and Lloyd 1988), and key word signing does not require any equipment. Furthermore, signs can be introduced at a very early stage of development, as in studies on early intervention with children with Down syndrome (Johansson 1988, Layton and Savino 1990, Launonen 1996). Signing with these children mostly means adding signed key words to speech-based communication. The signs used in this form of communication are picked from the deaf sign language. However, using a key word strategy does not mean the same as using sign language. The deaf sign language has its own grammar that makes it impossible to use parallel to talking with a spoken grammar. For a child who hears and understands spoken language this will always be the main source of information, even if s/he does not communicate with speech or uses only a few words of spoken language. Therefore a parallel use of signed key words together with speech is preferable, with some exceptions. In some cases, as for example with some autistic children, experience suggests that the child better benefits from first the spoken message and then the key signs, or vice versa (Carr *et al.* 1978). For a child who does not speak, signs can serve as an alternative to spoken language, and for a child with limited speech ability it will augment expressive communication. Signs might for some children be an initial modality of expression but later be dropped as speech develops (Johansson 1987). There are also indications that the combination of signs and speech may enhance the child's understanding of the spoken word and thus help the child to obtain information and improve cognitive skills (Johansson 1990, Launonen 1996).

Even if manual signs have proved to have a positive impact on early communication development for many children with disabilities, there might still be resistance from parents who are advised to start signing with their child. It puts demands on the family to learn and to use signs. If the parents feel that they do understand their child already, it is hard to see the need for signs. Another reason could be that it does not feel natural to use signs with a child who hears and maybe also understands spoken language. Finally there might be a fear that spoken language will be delayed if another communicative modality is introduced, though signs in fact often have the opposite effect on speech development. To overcome the obstacles mentioned it is important for parents to understand the reasons for manual sign use with the child with a disability. Thus, an important task for the professional is to provide explanations, knowledge and skills to parents.

Even though the introduction of manual signs is a part of many diagnosis-specific interventions (*e.g.* for children with Down syndrome), it is not the diagnosis *per se* that leads to this AAC intervention. Compared to speech, signs have characteristics that may facilitate communication and language development (Martinsen and von Tetzchner 1996). Signs are visual, while speech is auditory, and many children with disabilities have better use of visual perception than of hearing perception. The spoken word is more dynamic than the sign, which means that as soon as the word is said, it is gone, and there is a very limited time for perception. A sign, on the other hand, can be produced at a slower rate and to some degree extended when produced without being distorted. There are also differences in the motor skills required for speech versus sign production. Use of the mouth and tongue is far more complicated than use of the hands and fingers. A child with learning disabilities may need assistance for learning how to produce a word. It is then easier for the adult to shape, prompt and cooperate in sign production than in speech production. Also, the level of abstraction may differ. Manual signs are cognitively easier to produce at an early level of development. Many signs are more iconic than the corresponding spoken word, *i.e.* there is a resemblance between the sign and the concept it refers to (*e.g.* the sign for drinking shows the action of drinking). For spoken words there are no such links between the word and the referent, which probably explains why a small child at an early stage of language development refers to the concept 'car' with the sound of a car instead of saying the word.

However, there is one big advantage of speech compared to signs—as a communication model speech is far more frequently used than signs. Expressive language is not to be expected if there is not a lot of language input. Children need to see others use signs before they will produce them in communication. That is, persons in the family environment have to use signs to a greater extent, and for some time, before the child can be expected to respond to them.

Signs can be incorporated into any interactive activities normally carried out with a child such as mealtimes, play, story book reading, nursing and of course outdoor activities. There are different approaches to the introduction of signs, with some practitioners advocating that only a limited number of signs should be introduced at a time and used frequently in specific situations before the sign vocabulary is increased. Others have a more 'natural' view on signs and recommend that any spoken utterances should be accompanied by key signs, to make sign a natural communication mode. To increase functional communication skills it is quite obvious that an appropriate sign should be presented whenever it is needed. This incidental approach is recommended by most interventionists, but it puts demands on the environment to have an appropriate sign vocabulary. This might not be as big a problem as it may seem. Knowing only a limited number of signs often has the effect that the speech is simplified and the same kind of expressions are used repeatedly, which in fact may enhance the child's comprehension. A lack of knowledge about a certain sign that seems important in a certain situation can often be repaired afterwards. Signing to the child is one part of signed communication. The other part is helping the child to produce signs by her/himself. A few signs at a time might be selected. When selecting the first vocabulary it is important that the signs are useful and highly motivating to the child. These could be signs for a desired activity or object but could also be signs of more general use like the sign for 'more', 'look' or 'mine'. Teaching signs in a natural context, or milieu teaching, is a concept that stresses the importance of following the child's lead or interest (Kaiser *et al.* 1992). Often it is the child's inability to make specific demands and requests that motivates the environment to implement signs. However, it is just as important to guide the child to use signs with different communicative functions, *i.e.* for joint attention when looking in a picture book or playing together.

To summarize, signs used in combination with speech have several advantages both for the child (low demands on cognitive and motor abilities, higher iconicity increase understanding) and the interaction (lower pace, shorter sentences, etc.). Parents need to be informed of these advantages as well as guided in the use of signs. This is only possible if the intervention is based on the parents' perceived needs in communicating with their child.

MOVING FROM NONVERBAL, UNAIDED COMMUNICATION TO AIDED COMMUNICATION

Aided communication, that is, using a communication board, a speaking device or other physical aid to communicate, is most often used by non-speaking children with physical disabilities who have a limited capability to use manual signs (von Tetzchner and Martinsen, 1996, van Balkom and Welle Donker-Gimbrère 1996). However, aided communication can be used by children who need AAC for different purposes (Beukelman and Mirenda 1992).

Aided communication can vary both along a form dimension (*i.e.* from objects representing activities to arbitrary symbols for concepts) and a content dimension (*i.e.* from communicating about experiences, persons and objects in the 'here and now' situation to communicating about abstract concepts) (Granlund 1993).

The most basic form of aided communication is to use real objects (Basil and Soro-Camats 1996). They are often used with children at an early developmental age, who do not understand spoken language and/or need to be prepared for what is going to happen next (Beukelman and Mirenda 1992). Objects can be used in a naturalistic setting or in a highly structured one. The mother may show the child a spoon when it is time to eat, shoes when they are going out, a duck before a bath, and a teddy when it is time for bed. This strategy builds on the existing routines in the family, and does not require much adaptation of their daily life. Real objects can also be used in a schedule that provides a structure for the child's day. This is widely used with autistic children, but many other children also benefit from this approach. Schedules can be organized in different ways, but it is common to use boxes for the objects or to hang them in the right order on the wall. The child goes to the box/wall before the activity, takes the object and brings it along into the activity, and after the activity puts the object back into the box or onto the wall, to signal that the activity is ended. As the child develops, the objects may be replaced by photos, pictures, graphic symbols or written words. This approach makes high demands on the family to structure their day, but for a family with an autistic child this may be considered worth the effort, if the result is a more amenable child.

So far, we have looked at aided communication only as a tool for comprehension, but it can also be used for expression and social interaction (Beukelman and Mirenda 1992, Martinsen and von Tetzchner 1996). The most important communication goals for young children are to express needs and wants, and to achieve social closeness (Light 1997b). Sharing information and fulfilling the established conventions for social etiquette gain importance as the child grows older.

To be able to express her/his wants and needs, the child can be taught to make choices. A basic requirement for this approach is that the child can express acceptance and rejection. This is not identical to being able to indicate yes and no, which requires far more understanding (Beukelman and Mirenda 1992). Opportunities for choices between objects can be provided in many situations during the day, using the natural objects at hand. The parents may hold two objects in front of the child and ask which one s/he wants. At mealtimes, the child may choose between drinks, what to have in a sandwich, what fruit to eat, etc. Children who can choose between two objects, can move on to choose between several objects and/or photos, pictures and graphic symbols. For this approach to be successful, it is important that the parents and professionals work closely together to identify the child's interests and activities, and to find frequently occurring situations where making choices will fulfil a functional purpose (Calculator and Jorgensen 1991).

A simple diary or communication book can be an important communication tool (Rydeman 1990), and provide a child with a means of sharing information. In this book remnants from the child's day can be used as a basis for communicative interactions. The remnants can be real objects, or parts of objects, leftovers such as a brand label from an apple, a stick from an ice-cream or lollipop, or a ticket or other things that may remind the child of an event s/he has taken part in. Also photos, drawings or graphic symbols can be used. If the child attends a preschool or school, the book may be used as a communication book where the parents and staff write about the child's day, but where the child can tell her/his own story by pointing to the pictures or objects. It can also help the child to set the topic for a conversation (Beukelman and Mirenda 1992). For autistic children, the diary may be a logical continuation of the cues in the box or on the wall, and many children grow very attached to their books. They may read them over and over again to themselves, but also use them to tell others about things that are important to them.

If it is incorporated into the daily routines, a simple voice output device can provide many opportunities for a child to take part in family interactions (Beukelman and Mirenda 1992). There are several devices on the market that are easy for children to operate and for the parents or siblings to record new messages into. When the child presses a button, the device speaks a message. It can make it possible for a child to say thanks after a meal, wish the parents good night, greet guests that come to the house, or in other ways share the same social etiquette that is expected of other members of the family. The device may not make it easier for the parents to understand what the child wants, but it can make it possible for the child to start a conversation, deliver information, take part in storytelling or just simply get heard. If they use their imagination, the parents can give the non-speaking child a lot of new opportunities, and children often love the reactions they get from others to what they say with these devices.

Sometimes parents seem to regard aided communication as something that is in the way of natural communication (Basil and Soro-Camats 1996), or as an educational tool, instead of a means for communication (von Tetzchner and Martinsen 1996). This may be due to limitations in the graphic communication system itself, such as lack of speed or limited vocabulary (von Tetzchner and Martinsen 1996), or it may reflect the fact that the graphic system is not developed as a means to solve a communicative problem for the family and child.

In order for a solution to make a real difference to the child's life, it has to build on a consensus between the parents and the professionals about what has to be done, and why. This is especially important when more complex aided communication systems are introduced, such as communication boards and speech output devices that can hold many words and messages. They have to be based on a thorough knowledge of the child, the activities s/he takes part in during the day, her/his interests, and the communication partners. For example, recent research (Fallon and Light 2000, Tomasello 2000) has revealed that young children with and without disability organize concepts and linguistic schemata around concrete events and activities rather than around adult-like linguistic categories such as nouns and verbs. These new findings present significant problems for clinicians using formal grammatical categories as analytical tools in designing interventions.

DEVELOPING A FLEXIBLE COMPREHENSIVE COMMUNICATION INTERVENTION APPROACH
The focus for communication intervention for a child and her/his family will vary over time.

Variations will be seen in the goals for intervention as well as in the methods of achieving them. It is therefore important to stress the multidimensional aspects of communication, with regard to both the form and content of intervention.

The content of interaction and interactional patterns are important dimensions. AAC strategies are means for the child with a disability to interact in a more efficient way with persons in the environment. The ultimate outcome is always a high degree of participation in society and self-determination (Wehmeyer 1998). Communicative behaviours tend to be used for the same function and in the same interactional roles as they are taught (Reichle 1997). For this reason it is important that the desired use of the skills taught is considered by both professionals and parents. Examples of AAC outcomes that reflect a greater participation in interaction (Calculator 1999) include increased success of initiations, increased number of messages directed to the child, and increased variety of partners with whom the child exchanges messages.

Another important content dimension is the form for communication. Aided and unaided communication modes are not mutually exclusive, but rather can supplement each other. A child who uses manual signs as the primary means of communication may benefit from using a communication aid when talking to strangers who might not understand her/his signs. A child who uses a high-tech voice output communication aid cannot take it everywhere, and such a device cannot meet all her/his communication needs. The basic communication tools are still eye contact, facial expression, gestures, vocalization and, often, some manual signs (Heim and Baker-Mills 1996). They are fast and they are always there. Thus different kinds of AAC strategies may be combined in a total communication approach.

The form of communication intervention determines the degree of explicit training and the methods used (von Tetzchner 1997). The dimension extends from stimulating naturally occurring interaction (*i.e.* using implicit learning strategies) to highly structured training sessions with explicit goals for each session (*i.e.* explicit training strategies). Parents of young children have a tendency to be more training-focused and to more frequently adopt the role of trainer than do parents of older children (Adolfsson and Resare 1999). Parents of older children tend to define the communicative problem of the children in terms of interaction rather than language development and stress the importance of a natural context. Probably the efficacy of implicit training strategies for training the use of voice output systems and language acquisition has been underestimated. Sevcik *et al.* (1999) in an intervention study concerning children with severe to profound disabilities, report that the use of naturally occurring interaction contexts and implicit training strategies both increases the use of voice output systems and enhances language acquisition.

Another important dimension in communication intervention, especially if implicit training strategies are used, is the adaptation of the communicative environment. In a hybrid model for parent-implemented language intervention, Kaiser (1993) has identified three components of environmental adaptation: (1) environmental arrangement, (2) responsive interaction, and (3) milieu teaching. Regarding environmental arrangement, parents are taught to select toys and materials that are of interest to the child, to engage in play with the toys, to match and elicit the child's play schemes, and to set up situations designed to elicit interaction (*e.g.* to place a desired object out of reach). Responsive interaction includes following the child's lead, facilitating turn taking, etc. Finally, in relatively few milieu teaching episodes embedded in the environmental arrangements and responsive interaction, parents are taught to teach elaborated use of AAC in response to child initiations.

Conclusion

Communication intervention is one of the main means for supporting, within the family context, the development of children at risk of not developing speech. AAC intervention must support both the child and the family environment to be functional. The role of parents is central both in intervention decisions and in implementing intervention. For this reason professionals must perceive parents as competent collaborators in a mutual learning process that extends over long time periods. The focus and goals of this learning process are value-based and will vary over time, which necessitates a flexible stance from professionals.

REFERENCES

Adolfsson, M., Resare, E. (1999) *Samarbete en Förutsättning*. Västerås, Sweden: Mälardalen University.
Affleck, G., Tennen, H., Rowe, J., Roscher, B., Walker, L. (1989) 'Effects of formal support on mother's adaptation to hospital to home transition of high-risk infants: the benefits and costs of helping.' *Child Development*, **60**, 488–501.
Bailey, D., Simeonsson, R. (1988) *Family Assessment in Early Intervention*. London: Merrill.
Barnard, K., Kelly, J. (1990) 'Assessment of parent–child interaction.' *In:* Meisels, S.J., Shonkoff, J.P. (Eds.) *Handbook of Early Childhood Intervention*. New York: Cambridge University Press, pp. 278–302.
Basil, C., Soro-Camats, E. (1996) 'Supporting graphic language aqusition by a girl with multiple impairments.' *In:* von Tetzchner, S., Hygum Jensen, M. (Eds.) *Augmentative and Alternative Communication – European Perspectives*. London: Whurr, pp. 270–291.
Beukelman, D.R., Mirenda, P. (1992) *Augmentative and Alternative Communication. Management of Severe Communication Disorders in Children and Adults*. London: Paul H. Brookes.
Björck-Åkesson, E. (1993) *Communicative Interaction Between Young Non-speaking Children with Physical Disabilities and their Parents*. Jönköping, Sweden: Jönköping University Press.
—— Granlund, M., Olsson, C. (1996) 'Collaborative problem solving in communication intervention.' *In:* von Tetzchner, S., Hygum Jensen, M. (Eds.) *Augmentative and Alternative Communication – European Perspectives*. London: Whurr, pp. 324–341.
—— Brodin, J., Fälth, I-B. (1997) *Åtgärder–Samspel–Kommunikation*. Rockneby, Sweden: WRP International.
—— Granlund, M., Simeonsson, R. (2000) 'Assessment philosophies and practicies in Sweden.' *In:* Guralnick, M. (Ed.) *Interdisciplinary Clinical Assessment of Young Children with Developmental Disabilities*. London: Brookes, pp. 391–412.
Brodin, J. (1991) *Att Tolka Barns Signaler*. Stockholm: Stockholm University.
Calculator, S. (1999) 'AAC outcomes for children and youths with severe disabilities: when seeing is believing.' *Augmentative and Alternative Communication*, **15**, 4–12.
—— Jorgensen, C.M. (1991) 'Integrating AAC instruction into regular education settings: Expounding on best practices.' *Augmentative and Alternative Communication*, **7**, 204–214.
Carr, E.G., Binkoff, J.A., Kologinsky, E., Eddy, M. (1978) 'Acquisition of sign language by autistic children. I. Expressive labelling.' *Journal of Applied Behavior Analysis*, **11**, 459–501.
Dunst, C., Trivette, C., Deal, A. (1994) *Supporting and Strengthening Families*. Cambridge: Brookline.
Fallon, K., Light, J. (2000) 'The semantic organization patterns of young children: Implications for AAC.' *In: Conference Proceedings – Ninth Biennial Conference of the International Society for Augmentative and Alternative Communication, August, Washington DC, USA*, pp. 431–433.
Gallagher, J. (1990) 'The family as a focus for intervention.' *In:* Meisels, S., Shonkoff, J. (Eds.) *Handbook of Early Childhood Intervention*. Cambridge: Cambridge University Press, pp. 540–559.
Gallimore, R., Weisner, T., Bernheimer, L., Guthrie, D., Nihara, K. (1993) 'Family responses to children with developmental delays.' *American Journal on Mental Retardation*, **98**, 185–206.
—— Coots, J., Weisner, T., Garnier, H., Guthrie, D. (1996) 'Family responses to children with early developmental

delays. II: Accomodation intensity and activity in early and middle childhood.' *American Journal on Mental Retardation,* **101**, 215–232.

Granlund, M. (1993) *Communicative Competence in Persons with Profound Mental Retardation. Acta Universitatis Upsaliensis.* Stockholm: Almquist & Wiksell.

—— Olsson, C. (1998) *Familjen och Habiliteringen.* Stockholm: ALA Research Foundation.

—— —— (1999) 'Communication intervention for pre-symbolic communicators.' *Augmentative and Alternative Communication,* **15**, 25–37.

—— Björck-Åkesson, E., Brodin, J., Olsson, C. (1995) 'Communication intervention for persons with profound disabilities: A Swedish perspective.' *Augmentative and Alternative Communication,* **11**, 49–59.

—— Björck-Åkesson, E., Sandell, C. (1998) *Ekokulturell Intervju – en Pilotstudie.* Västerås, Sweden: Mälardalen University.

Heim, M., Baker-Mills, A. (1996) 'Early development of symbolic communication and linguistic complexity through augmentative and alternative communication.' *In:* von Tetzchner, S., Hygum Jensen, M. (Eds.) *Augmentative and Alternative Communication – European Perspectives.* London: Whurr, pp. 232–248.

Johansson, I. (1987) *Tecken – en Genväg till Tal. Down Syndrom: Språk och Tal nr. 7.* Umeå University, Dept of Phonetics. publication 28.

—— (1988) *Språkutveckling hos Handikappade Barn.* Lund, Sweden: Studentlitteratur.

—— (1990) 'Contributions of language to cognitive development.' *Paper presented at the Fourth Biennial Conference of ISAAC, Stockholm.*

Kaiser, A.P. (1993) 'Parent-implemented language intervention: an environmental systems perspective.' *In:* Kaiser, A., Gray, D. (Eds.) *Enhancing Children's Communication: Research Foundations for Intervention.* London: Paul Brookes, pp. 63–84.

—— Yoder, P.J., Keetz, A. (1992) 'Evaluating milieu teaching.' *In:* Warren, S.F., Reichle, J. (Eds.) *Causes and Effects in Communication and Language Intervention.* London: Paul Brooks, pp. 9–47.

Kangas, K., Lloyd, L. (1988) 'Early cognitive skill prerequisites to augmentative and alternative communication use: What are we waiting for?' *Augmentative and Alternative Communication,* **4**, 211–221.

Ketelaar, M., Vermeer, A., Helders, P., Hart, H. (1998) 'Parental participation in intervention programs for children with cerebral palsy.' *Topics in Early Childhood Special Education,* **18**, 108–117.

Kiresuk, T., Smith, A., Cardillo, J. (1994) *Goal Attainment Scaling, Applications, Theory and Measurement.* London: Lawrence Earlbaum.

Lagerheim, B. (1988) *Att Utvecklas med Handikapp.* Stockholm: Nordstedt Förlag.

Launonen, K. (1996) 'Enhancing communication skills of children with Down syndrome: Early use of manual signs.' *In:* von Tetzchner, S., Hygum Jensen, M. (Eds.) *Augmentative and Alternative Communication – European Perspectives.* London: Whurr, pp. 213–231.

Layton, T.L., Savino, M.A. (1990) 'Acquiring a communication system by sign and speech in a child with Down syndrome: A longitudinal investigation.' *Child Language Teaching and Therapy,* **6**, 59–76.

Leskinen, M. (1994) *Family in Focus.* Jyväskylä, Finland: Jyväskylä University Press.

Light, J. (1997a) 'Communication is the essence of human life: Reflections on communicative competence.' *Augmentative and Alternative Communication,* **13**, 61–70.

—— (1997b) 'Let's go starfishing: Reflections on the contexts of language learning for children who used aided AAC.' *Augmentative and Alternative Communication,* **13**, 158–171.

—— McNaughton, D., Parnes, P. (1986) *A Protocol for the Assessment of Communication Interaction Skills of Non-speaking Severely Handicapped Adults and their Facilitators.* Toronto: Hugh McMillan Centre.

Martinsen, H., von Tetzchner, S. (1996) 'Situating augmentative and alternative communication intervention.' *In:* von Tetzchner, S., Hygum Jensen, M. (Eds.) *Augmentative and Alternative Communication – European Perspectives.* London: Whurr, pp 37–48.

McCollum, J., Hemmeter, M-L. (1997) 'Parent–child interaction intervention when children have disabilities.' *In:* Guralnick, M. (Ed.) *The Effectiveness of Early Intervention.* Baltimore: Paul H. Brookes, pp. 549–576.

Parette, H., Brotherson, M. (1996) 'Family participation in assistive technology assessment for young children with mental retardation and developmental disabilities.' *Education and Training in Mental Retardation and Developmental Disabilities,* **31**, 29–43.

Reichle, J. (1997) 'Communication intervention with persons who have severe disabilities.' *Journal of Special Education,* **31**, 110–134.

Roll-Pettersson, L. (1997) *Föräldrar till Skolbarn med Begåvningshandikapp Berättar om Sina Känslomässiga Upplevelser.* Stockholm: ALA Research Foundation.

—— Granlund, M., Steénson, A-L. (1999) 'Familjers behov – Lärares behov.' *In:* Granlund, M., Steénson,

A-L., Roll-Pettersson, L., Björck-Åkesson, E., Sundin, M., Kylén, A. (Eds.) *Elever med Flera Funktionsnedsättningar i Särskolan – Utbildningens Effekter och Effektivitet.* Stockholm: ALA Research Foundation, pp. 105–180.

Rydeman, B. (1990) *Tala med Tecken.* Halmstad, Sweden: Habiliteringen, Landstinget Halland.

Sameroff, A., Fiese, B. (1990) 'Transactional regulation and early intervention.' *In:* Meisels, S., Shonkoff, J. (Eds.) *Handbook of Early Childhood Intervention.* Cambridge: Cambridge University Press, pp. 119–149.

Sevcik, R., Romski, M., Adamson, L. (1999) 'Measuring AAC intervention for individuals with severe developmental disabilities.' *Augmentative and Alternative Communication,* **15**, 38–44.

Tomasello, M. (2000) 'The item-based nature of children's early syntactic development.' *Trends in Cognitive Science,* **4**, 156–163.

van Balkom, H., Welle Donker-Gimbrère, M. (1996) 'A psycholinguistic approach to graphic language use.' *In:* von Tetzchner, S., Hygum Jensen, M. (Eds.) *Augmentative and Alternative Communication – European Perspectives.* London: Whurr, pp. 153–170.

Wehmeyer, M. (1998) 'Self-determination and individuals with significant disabilities: Examining meanings and misinterpretations.' *Journal of the Association for Persons with Severe Handicaps,* **23**, 5–16.

von Tetzchner, S. (1997) *Theoretical Perspectives on Language Development and Language Intervention.* Helsinki: Sillala på Bron Seminari.

—— Hygum Jensen, M. (1996) 'Introduction.' *In:* von Tetzchner, S., Hygum Jensen, M. (Eds.) *Augmentative and Alternative Communication – European Perspectives.* London: Whurr, pp. 1–18.

—— Martinsen, H. (1996) 'Words and strategies: Conversations with young children who use aided language.' *In:* von Tetzchner, S., Hygum Jensen, M. (Eds.) *Augmentative and Alternative Communication – European Perspectives.* London: Whurr, pp. 65–88.

6
SUPPORTING CHILDREN USING AUGMENTATIVE AND ALTERNATIVE COMMUNICATION IN SCHOOL

Sally Millar

> "Language is central to learning. It provides the main tool for teaching and learning and, by experiencing language for these purposes, children's language develops further. Through active participation and through interaction with people and with their environment, children learn to make sense of their world."
>
> Martin and Miller (1999)

Much of every child's development—educational, social, emotional and cultural—takes place through communication. This chapter—without going into practical details of how to go about providing appropriate support on a day-to-day classroom basis—suggests key areas of policy, planning and practice that make for educational environments supportive to children who need to use AAC in order to fulfil their communication and educational potential. The key to successful support of children using AAC is not just about AAC in itself, or about individual AAC users. It is more to do with 'systems issues', such as how schools organize themselves, how they organize provision to meet the individual support needs of pupils, how AAC is perceived in schools, and who takes responsibility for supporting AAC.

Special educational needs

Children need functional communication skills in order to interact with their environment, to express themselves and to make social relationships. They need to develop some language in order to participate in, and benefit fully from, the educational process. Severe speech, language and communication impairments are undoubtedly a major barrier to the development of thinking, reasoning, remembering and learning. Additionally, many children with communication difficulties are likely to have further impairments of physical, motor, sensory, perceptual or social function, and/or other learning difficulties, giving rise overall to what educational agencies call 'special educational needs' (SEN).

By definition, all children with special educational needs require effective special educational support. Specific details of policy and provision differ from country to country. This chapter uses examples mainly from UK educational systems; readers from other countries will be able to apply the principles to the situation in their own settings. In the UK, as in many countries, the right to effective educational provision for children with special needs is enshrined in national legislation [for example: in England and Wales, the Education Act 1980; in the USA, the Education for all Handicapped Children Act 1975, renamed as the Individuals with Disabilities Education Act (IDEA) 1990].

Thomson *et al.* (1995) constructively reframed the issue of special educational needs as one of *educational support needs*, emphasizing different levels of support needs and the steps that might be taken by schools and other agencies to meet these needs, rather than defining individual children by their medical diagnosis, disability or 'problems'.

The need to use AAC represents a special category of educational support need that may be obscured by all the child's other educational support needs (access ramps, transport, nursing care, etc.), or that may be ignored because it is poorly understood. To highlight the issue, it might help to 'translate' AAC into educational terminology, as a particular type of *'communication support need'*.

COMMUNICATION SUPPORT NEEDS

The high level of communication support needs of school students using AAC is commonly underestimated, at the level of policy and funding of provision. This is probably due to the lack of reliable data about how many children within the school system need to use AAC, the lack of clear information and understanding of the nature of AAC support needs, and the lack of evaluative evidence about what types of support work best and how these should be delivered. AAC is a new field, and more research evidence is needed.

Broadly, the communication support needs of children requiring AAC are likely to include:

- intensive and ongoing teaching, therapy and support input, to promote the development of social understanding, personal communication and language
- introduction of a low-tech communication system tailored to the child's needs, at as early an age as possible
- provision of good quality materials giving access to the curriculum through an appropriate medium (*e.g.* in pictures and symbols)
- additional staff time and equipment, for the creation and use of such materials
- additional school staffing to provide classroom support
- ongoing input from specialized professional(s) to provide:
  - assessment for appropriate high-tech AAC system(s), and regular reassessment
  - introduction of AAC
  - ongoing teaching and day-to-day practice in the use of AAC systems
  - ongoing training and support in AAC for teaching and support staff in school
- development of a consistent approach among all those working with the AAC user in school
- designing appropriate individual educational programmes (IEPs), setting appropriate targets and developing appropriate teaching programmes for pupils using AAC
- integrating the use of AAC systems into all classroom activities and into all IEP/curriculum-led teaching and learning
- innovative and imaginative classroom practice to ensure provision of (specially engineered, if necessary) communication opportunities

- special educational approaches to support the acquisition of literacy
- additional staff time for transdisciplinary joint planning and curriculum development, to provide integration of communication and language with general educational targets and tasks
- integration of AAC use with use of personalized computer-based aids to allow for access to the full curriculum and to support writing
- funding support for AAC device(s) and computers for classroom work
- planning for continuity, and providing training and support in AAC across students' transitions—*e.g.* nursery to primary; class to class, every year; primary to secondary; secondary to school-leaving.

This is an impressive and challenging list; it is clear that these needs will not be met effectively through an ad hoc approach. There are major implications regarding policy, planning, funding, interdisciplinary collaboration, training and practice development.

BEST PRACTICE?

Unfortunately, 'best practice' in AAC support, from the perspective of specialists in AAC (Johnson *et al.* 1996, Glennen and DeCoste 1997, Beukelman and Mirenda 1998), is not necessarily reflected in schools. In many cases, expensive high-tech AAC devices are purchased but not used due to inappropriate assessment recommendations (Phillips and Zhao 1993) or, most commonly, to lack of appropriate training and support (ICAC 1995, Murphy *et al.* 1996). AAC systems are often taught but not used outside the therapy setting (Murphy *et al.* 1995). The current reality is that in many schools effective teaching and support of communication skills and AAC use is severely compromised by (amongst other things), the following:

- limited levels of school staff awareness, experience and training in the impact of medical conditions on the development of speech and language, and in augmentative communication
- in the UK, and perhaps elsewhere, the absence of any statutory requirement for appropriately qualified teachers to provide for communication needs specifically (in contrast to statutory requirements relating to teachers of children with visual and hearing impairments)
- over-reliance on untrained special needs assistants/aides to implement and support students' AAC programmes
- school staff's lack of time
- pressure upon staff to give priority to other curricular aims and care needs
- limited funding availability for the purchase of AAC devices and for the support staffing necessary to implement and support its use
- shortfall in appropriate speech and language therapy input
- barriers created by school staff attitudes (*e.g.* a desire to 'normalize' children, evidenced by a reluctance to have aids to communication)
- inadequate understanding of, or commitment to, planning and support at times of student transition, *e.g.* from primary to secondary school.

DIFFERENT CULTURES

The worlds of AAC and schools are two quite distinct 'cultures', each with different philosophical and theoretical roots, and each with a different focus. Pioneering work in the relatively new field of AAC has been dominated by specialist speech and language therapists, whose training and roots 'traditionally' lie within the medical domain (as do, in many cases, their day-to-day employment conditions). Education has its own paradigms and terminologies, and teachers' work in practice is shaped by educational structures and procedures (many determined by government edict) and by the ethos and hierarchy of individual schools. Priorities are different; schools and classes are essentially 'group cultures' where meeting the needs of *all* children is a paramount aim, whereas the focus in health and therapy (and parents, naturally) is on the needs of the individual child. Providing effective support for students who use AAC in classrooms means, in effect, trying to bring these two different cultures closer together.

DIFFERENT TYPES OF SCHOOL PLACEMENT

Before the child gets to school, there will be discussions between parents and professionals as to the most appropriate educational placement. The choice will generally be between:
- special (self-contained) school
- special class or unit within, or attached to, a mainstream school (offering some degree of integration of students at certain points in the daily or weekly timetable)
- mainstream school classroom with support from specialist teachers and/or special needs assistants, as required.

(Different political, cultural or geographical settings may offer slightly different options or different types of funding structures and degrees of support and integration within these broad options.)

Communication and language play such a major role in a child's cognitive and educational development that they should be considered as key indicators at times of review of school placement.

The dominant social and political trend in developed countries is toward *inclusion*— education in the *least restrictive environment*—*e.g.* in the USA, the Individuals with Disabilities Education Act 1990, and guidelines of the UN (1993) and UNESCO (1994). The term 'inclusion' is sometimes misinterpreted as meaning 'all children should be in their local mainstream school', whereas in reality a range of alternative types of provision and support are needed, to avoid 'maindumping' (Wylie 2000), and to meet different students' needs and parental concerns. As Blamires (1999) highlights, there are at least three dimensions to educational inclusion: physical, cognitive and social. Resolving physical access and medical support issues in any type of setting by no means guarantees that social and cognitive needs are adequately catered for. Social integration may sometimes be at the expense of a student's other support needs (*e.g.* specialized communication and education issues).

There is no 'best' placement for an AAC user—each case should be considered in the light of individual circumstances and the range of educational provision available. The advantage of mainstream settings may lie in access to a full educational curriculum and especially in social contact with a peer group providing 'normal' communication role models and a link with the local community (often a priority for parents). However, there is also day-to-day evidence that the highly specialist nature of the communication support needs of AAC users—and the huge time demands of such support—may be 'a bridge too far' for many mainstream schools (especially at secondary level), even though they are able to cope well with students with physical difficulties alone.

Compromise attempts, such as 'split placements' are generally a poor solution; the child often spends a large part of the school day 'in transit', and the staff in neither setting have time to gain in-depth knowledge of the child's communication system. Neither school may perceive itself as having responsibility for meeting the child's communication support needs.

Special schools may offer more therapy input and a higher staff–student ratio overall. In the best of scenarios, they may offer access to a valuable concentration of staff experience and expertise with AAC. However, AAC is a specialism even within special settings, and not all special schools are AAC-experienced or AAC-friendly. Smaller, local special units and classes may also have problems; many are coping with a hugely diverse range of special needs within one small group of children—staff cannot be experts in all specialisms at once. AAC and education cultures may therefore be as far apart from each other in special as in mainstream settings.

Figures are available to indicate that in a number of countries the majority of children with special educational support needs are now in mainstream school settings, although the term 'mainstreaming' in many cases seems to refer to special units or classes within mainstream schools, rather than full-time schooling in regular classrooms [England, 60% (DfEE 1999); USA, 75% (OSEP 2000); New Zealand, 54% (Wylie 2000)]. There are no figures available to show how many of these are children who use AAC (or who might need to use AAC, though they have not yet been provided with it). Certainly the overall number of children using AAC in mainstream schools is gradually increasing. This poses major challenges, in that AAC services and the training of teachers and other professionals in basic AAC issues and skills now need to be provided 'across the board' and not just targeted at a few specialist schools.

MODELS OF PROVISION
Medical model of support?
Communication is not a 'within-person' skill but a dynamic, interactive and social process. A 'medical model' approach to communication—one that focuses narrowly on a skill-based view of an individual child who is referred, assessed, diagnosed, then 'prescribed' an AAC system and a programme of treatment, which is then delivered to the child in a clinical setting outside the classroom—is likely to be the least effective model of support for an AAC user.

Until recently the traditional approach of staff in many schools was to perceive communication issues and the development of AAC as the exclusive province of speech and language therapists; however, it is now increasingly recognized that relying entirely on non-educationalists and/or outside specialists is not a viable approach (Calculator and Jorgensen 1991). On a pragmatic level, speech and language therapy services are seriously understaffed and overstretched in many areas, and not all speech and language therapists have specialist AAC knowledge. Although speech and language therapists can meet some of the communication support needs of pupils, they cannot take responsibility for meeting AAC users' curricular and educational needs (Reid *et al.* 1996, Wright 1996).

School-based model of support
A more effective model will be to try to develop a supportive school environment that:
- accepts that the development and use of children's language and communication skills is an educational issue and ultimately the responsibility of *school* staff;
- includes individual specialist attention for AAC users within the curriculum and within day-to-day classroom practice situations (rather than as an occasional and separate 'add-on');
- incorporates work on language and communication goals for AAC students in natural, functional and social contexts, rather than in artificially created one-to-one situations.

Within this model, speech and language therapy input will be an important resource, although not the lead agency. An important factor contributing to successful AAC intervention will be the degree and quality of collaborative interdisciplinary working that is achieved at policy level as well as at day-to-day classroom working level (see below).

Developing a supportive school environment for AAC

> "Technology and augmentative communication systems are useless in enabling children to realize their potential without appropriate training and a supportive environment."
>
> (Burkhart 1993)

SETTING UP A FRAMEWORK
A supportive school environment for AAC will include development initiatives at a number of levels, some quite distant from the individual child. It may include the following:
- school policies on communication
- strategic use of official educational documentation such as individual student assessments, statements/records of need, individual educational programmes, action plans, school development plans, school staff training programmes, etc., with explicit and specific inclusion of AAC issues in all such documentation
- training in AAC for school staff
- effective collaborative interdisciplinary team-working
- appropriate assessment and provision procedures for AAC
- statutory funding for purchase of communication aid technology.

AAC POLICIES IN SCHOOLS
Before it will be supported, AAC has to be explicitly recognized and valued by schools as having equal but different status with natural speech (*i.e.* rather than being 'tacked on' as a low-status afterthought for a minority of 'failed' speakers). To this end, increasing numbers of schools are developing a written policy establishing access to communication as a human rights and equity issue for children, making an explicit whole-school commitment to AAC,

and laying down guidelines for good practice on the part of staff with regard to communication (Chinnery *et al.* 2001). Such a policy would cover areas including: definitions of AAC aims and approaches; goals for AAC users; assessment and management; curriculum; pupil experiences and activities; staffing and resources; and recording and evaluation. A good school policy should indicate who has responsibility for each specific area and will show where AAC planning integrates with wider curriculum development.

As an example, the policy of a school might include points such as:

- a recognition that the ability to communicate and to interact with the environment is fundamental to the development of the whole child
- all staff should be committed to enabling each student to optimize their potential for communication, interaction and access to educational opportunities through whatever means is most suitable for the individual
- AAC is the responsibility of the whole school
- AAC should be integrated throughout the curriculum
- each AAC user will have a written statement recording a summary of her/his AAC system and how s/he accesses it
- staff need to modify their own behaviour and communication in order to enable the augmented communicator to participate in the educational experiences
- staff need to develop and monitor their own listener skills
- staff should also use AAC systems in their interaction to promote the validity of the systems for communication and to establish a community of users
- students' needs and wants are not automatically fulfilled, therefore staff should recognize the importance of creating a need to communicate.

STRATEGIC USE OF EDUCATIONAL DOCUMENTATION; EXPLICIT INCLUSION OF AAC

As a general principle, in order to ensure that the AAC support needs of individual students are met in schools, it is first necessary to ensure that these are clearly and explicitly identified in all official *educational* documentation (medical and therapy records, which are generally confidential anyway, will not carry executive power within the education system).

The precise format of documentation will vary from country to country, although the content will be similar. In the UK, students will have a record/statement of special educational needs, and an individualized educational plan (IEP) (in the USA, the IEP performs both functions). Education authorities have a statutory duty to implement them, so these documents are potentially powerful tools. However, in research in London, Grove and Norwich (1997) found that AAC and appropriate provision to meet AAC support needs were rarely mentioned specifically. Communication support needs are often mentioned only very vaguely (*e.g.* "speech and language therapy to be provided as required", "X will benefit from the use of technology"), which has no power either to command allocation of resources or to guide practice.

To be useful in supporting AAC, specifics are necessary. Naming and costing technology at a highly detailed level is not appropriate, as both the child's needs and the technology available will change over time. It will be preferable to use a highly specific but generic formula such as: "Throughout his school career, Freddie will need ongoing exclusive access to a portable computer-based aid to personal communication with special input (touch screen) and output (voice output and hard copy print-out) facilities, with symbol-based software and pre-stored vocabulary."

In addition to technology needs, the child's requirement for ongoing support from AAC-trained staff will be emphasized. It is advisable to suggest a specific amount of specialist input that can be used as a benchmark, rather than simply putting "as required". Murphy *et al*. (1996) suggested that learning to use an AAC system is similar in some ways to mastering a foreign language—basic functional conversation skills may be acquired within about 200 hours, but true mastery requires many more hundreds of hours of teaching and learning, repetition and practice, over an extended period of time. Obviously, like foreign language learning, the more practice is obtained, the more fluent and confident the learner becomes. Two hundred hours works out at around one hour per school day, throughout the academic year—which could be split between speech and language therapy input and language, communication and AAC input delivered by other staff, partly in individual and partly in group settings.

Finally, official documents should record the need for reassessment of AAC needs every 1–3 years by a specialist centre or service, and for access to a loan bank of AAC equipment, to funding for purchase of AAC devices as recommended, and to ongoing technical support as required.

Creating a school environment that is generally supportive to AAC will inevitably have staffing, training and funding implications above and beyond the specific needs of particular students—for example, the need for AAC-related technology equipment purchases for school (such as computers with colour printers, for use by staff to create symbol-based materials, make back-ups of students' vocabularies etc.). Related to this, there will be a need for staff to have non-contact time in which to use this equipment, and to design and make such resources. Also, school staff will need ongoing training in AAC from AAC specialists. Mechanisms for securing funding for these ends will differ across countries/education authorities/schools, but a necessary feature, common to all, will be the explicit and specific inclusion of AAC in planning and budgeting at a general district/authority/school level in documents (such as, in the UK, the School Development Plan).

TRAINING IN AAC FOR SCHOOL STAFF

Soto (1997) found that class teachers' willingness to participate in interdisciplinary working and to develop and use innovatory teaching strategies with AAC users was strongly influenced by their own sense of self-efficacy. Many teachers had low confidence and self-esteem, and low expectations of their pupils, due to feelings of ignorance in the specialist area of AAC. This indicates a clear need for training and support from AAC specialists to *teachers*, as well as input to individual students.

Training will be pursued at several levels: awareness-raising on interaction and communication in general (Mendes and Rato 1996), language development and AAC, AAC and curriculum, AAC in the classroom, and technical aspects of specific AAC systems. Training in AAC cannot just be left informally in the hands of the school speech and language therapist, but needs to be actively managed/commissioned by school senior management (see also 'Joint Staff Development', below). At the very least, the school staff's formal training programme should include, each year:

- one or more AAC-related topic(s) on staff in-service calendar, for *all* school staff
- designated staff member(s) to attend an AAC conference/equipment exhibition, to keep up to date with new developments generally
- designated staff member(s) to attend specific training course(s) to ensure in-depth knowledge of specific AAC system(s) used by named student(s).

In order to create a supportive environment—rather than one specialized helper on whom the AAC student may become overdependent—and to cover staff changes and student progression from class to class, a whole range of school staff should be trained, including, importantly, special needs assistants. Training packs in AAC that can be delivered 'in-house' over a period of time, to groups of staff, will be a useful resource (McConachie and Pennington 1997).

The ideal goal is perhaps to see AAC included routinely alongside general language and communication issues at all levels of pre- and post-qualification professional education, rather than being kept separate. At a more specialist level, accredited postgraduate training in AAC (including distance learning components) is well established in a number of North American universities (*e.g.* University of Nebraska) but is just beginning in the UK (*e.g.* Manchester Metropolitan University).

COLLABORATIVE INTERDISCIPLINARY TEAM WORKING

As Downing (1999) contends, *"The responsibility of ensuring that all students have an effective means of communicating cannot fall to any one person."* The necessary support programmes for children using AAC require coordinated input from a range of people with different roles and skills, from preschool services, health, education, IT, social services, voluntary agencies and others. Successful support of AAC in schools depends on it, but professionals usually have no training in interdisciplinary collaboration and joint working (Lacey and Lomas 1993); supporting development of good practice in this area should be a government priority, to support inclusive educational policies.[1]

Pickles (1998) distinguishes between the support *team*, as those professionals working with the child on a regular hands-on basis within school (*e.g.* teaching, support and therapy staff), and the support *network*, as that team plus all the additional professionals from outside the immediate school setting who are involved less frequently (*e.g.* specialist teaching, medical, social work, rehabilitation engineering staff). We should also distinguish between those whose remit is to support the child directly, and those whose responsibility is strategic and managerial (*i.e.* supporting the school, to help them to support the child). The number of different professionals involved, whether regularly or intermittently, can easily run to 20 or more. However, the involvement of so many different professionals can often cause as many problems as it solves, if their input is not coordinated and synthesized into a unified approach.

It is strongly recommended that coordination of this process be an *educational*

---

[1]Inspectors of special schools (HMI, OFSTED) are increasingly aware of the importance of interdisciplinary team working between school staff and speech and language therapists (RCSLT 1996).

commitment. It is only when a school feels that it 'owns' the programme that effective AAC in education will be achieved for specific pupils. Each setting will require to identify:

- an agreed 'network coordinator', employed by the education service, whose role is to have an overview of planning and target setting, to monitor progress, and to ensure continuity for the AAC user. This person does not necessarily need to be around in class every day but must have the authority to follow up other network and team members, ensuring that recommendations and programmes are carried out, and fighting for resources, if necessary— for example, a member of school senior management. They will doubtless need and value close collaboration with the speech and language therapist(s) and AAC specialist(s)
- an agreed 'key person' in daily contact with the child and her/his other regular communication partners, able to direct and monitor daily events and deal with practical issues immediately, as they arise, and to feed back information to the network coordinator and other team members. This may be the class teacher in special schools and units, or the classroom special needs assistant in mainstream schools. They too will need ongoing input from the speech and language therapist(s).

In Scotland (Reid *et al.* 1996, Farmer and Reid 2001), the development of detailed written school level working practice agreements between schools and speech and language therapists is proving helpful in promoting closer and more effective collaborative practice.

AAC Coordinator or Communication Support Teacher
Some authorities and schools in the UK designate an 'AAC Coordinator' or 'Communication Support Teacher' with special responsibility for AAC. This role might include:

- overall monitoring of pupils' AAC programmes
- linking between areas of the curriculum for AAC users
- supporting classroom teachers and assistants in the knowledge and use of signing, symbols and communication technology in the classroom
- supporting pupils directly in class, and/or withdrawn for individual work, as required
- liaising with AAC and subject specialists, speech and language therapists, and other learning support staff
- managing a budget for purchase of items of communication technology, software upgrades, maintenance, repairs, etc., and keeping an inventory
- leading a programme to make information accessible to all students (for example, by ensuring the text of a school newsletter is supported by a system of picture symbols).

AAC specialists
AAC specialists need to consider how to make the most effective use of their skills. Cunningham and Davis (1985) suggest that the 'Transplant Model' (where experts' skills are transplanted into school staff and parents) and the 'Consumer Model' (two-way discussion between professionals and parents, about priorities, aims and methods) are more suitable working frameworks than an 'Expert Model'.

Johnson *et al.* (1996) have described a successful collaborative project where, rather than imposing a list of AAC techniques and educational competences to be attained by pupils, a mentor (the consultant expert in AAC in education) and a collaborator (a special education teacher) actively problem-solved together on personalizing a class-based programme to match the understandings and needs of the people within the system, sharing responsibility for all stages of the process. The result of this approach was a deep-rooted shift in the teacher's attitudes and teaching methods—an indirect rather than a direct form of support to the child using AAC. This sort of process takes time; it is realistic to think in terms of an ongoing contact throughout several school years.

Speech and language therapists

Speech and language therapists determine models of service delivery most suited to the classroom/school setting (RCSLT 1996). Because AAC work is so specialized and needs to be intensive, the hands-off 'therapist as consultant' model of therapy (devising programmes and leaving school staff to implement them), is likely to be inappropriate and ineffective. A hands-on collaborative approach is required. The American Speech–Language–Hearing Association (ASHA 1993) lists the main models of service delivery as:

- *collaborative consultation* (joint goal setting, curriculum development, adapting materials and teaching methods)
- *classroom-based integrated services* (team teaching and classroom facilitation)

(often both of the above models are used in conjunction, with emphasis on planning in the former, and on direct delivery of services in the latter)

- *pullout* [individually, or in small groups—particularly indicated for older students and when students are learning new skills—Clarke *et al.* (2001a)]
- *self-contained programmes* (losing relevance in today's inclusive climate).

ASHA recommends a therapy case-load of no more than 40 schoolchildren—and considerably less than that (8–12) for a time-intensive case load of all technology-dependent and/or medically fragile children. In addition to all the time required for liaison and joint planning with parents, school staff and other professionals, and for materials/technology development work, the input of therapy or specialist communication teaching needed by AAC users is likely to be more or less double that of speaking students. At least half an hour of focused AAC work, plus a total of at least another hour involving use of AAC in functional situations and educational activities, every day would be advisable.

Campaigning to expand support services and the strategic use of these is also important. Using AAC specialist or speech and language therapy time to create symbol resources, for example, is inefficient—better to spend the time teaching classroom teachers how to identify vocabulary needs and special needs assistants or therapy aides how to operate the software, so that they can design and create the resources between them.

Special needs assistants[1]

In many classrooms, although the class teacher has responsibility for the education of all of the children in the class, the special needs assistant (SNA) may have responsibility for implementing and supporting appropriate programmes for individual children with disabilities.

---

[1]Different countries will have different names for these important staff members and different training/qualification/salary/career development structures.

In practice, it is often the SNA who both manages and supports the child's AAC system in school, and who enables the child to use it in school. However, as a group, these important school staff members are often seriously undervalued and may miss out on training and paid time for joint planning work with teachers and therapists.

Enhancements to their status, working conditions, pay, support, and access to staff development opportunities are urgently required.

Joint staff development

The 'cascade' model of in-service development has been found ineffective in the area of severe communication disorders and AAC (Kersner and Wright 1996, SOEID 1996). A better model is one where teachers, speech and language therapists and, hopefully, SNAs can attend relevant training events *together*. Collaborative team working can also be supported by ongoing in-house staff development commitments such as weekly signing classes; ideally, *all* members of the team should take turns to lead joint staff development sessions in their particular area of work. Speech and language therapists need to learn more about the curriculum and education issues, just as teachers need to learn more about language development, communication issues and AAC.

To sum up, effective interdisciplinary collaborative working is likely to be characterized by the following:

- initiation, monitoring and support of collaborative practice at policy-making and senior management level
- clear and explicit mechanisms for coordination and communication
- timetabling that allows for non-contact time for joint planning and joint working between therapists, teachers and assistants
- opportunities and resources made available for joint training of teachers, therapists and other staff in AAC
- enhanced employment conditions and a career structure for SNAs.

Assessment and choice of AAC systems for school use

It is widely recognized (Kraat 1985, Light 1989) that the role of communication partners and the setting in which the individual is attempting to communicate have a powerful effect on the success—or otherwise—of AAC use. A common reason for AAC failure in schools is because an inappropriate assessment process has considered only half of the equation—the child alone—rather than evaluating the needs of *the developing child in the school context*, resulting in an inappropriate choice of AAC system.

There is no 'right' AAC system for a young school student, there are only systems that are 'workable' (or otherwise) within particular school settings. In general, a 'bottom up' approach, involving simple and practical systems, requiring little specialist training for staff, is more likely to be used in school classrooms. This may not be ideal, but can at least provide a solid and positive base of successful communicative interaction upon which can be built a more powerful system later. The 'top down' alternative might be too-early introduction of a complex high-tech AAC system that may be 'ideal' in theory but fail in practice and prove negative and demotivating all round.

It is now established (Murphy *et al.* 1995) that all AAC users are likely to use a number of different communication media simultaneously/interchangeably. These will include some elements of whole body gesture, facial expression, eye gaze and eye pointing, and vocalizations, as well as perhaps low and/or high-tech AAC systems. In the same way, in schools, children are likely to use all of these unaided systems plus pointing to symbol charts or books, and using a range of simple voice output devices and computers, as well as— possibly—a dedicated communication aid.

Additionally, influenced by school-based AAC practitioners (*e.g.* Goossens 1999, Burkhart 1993), specialists in early literacy development (Koppenhaver *et al.* 1993) and others (Millar 1998, Donnelly 2000), there is a growing trend in schools towards use of a variety of simple voice output AAC systems as general classroom resources, for use in a variety of ways in group activities, rather than use of a single AAC system as one particular child's 'special' aid. With this model, the dividing line between aids to learning and aids to communication becomes blurred. While this model is increasingly recognized as good practice in the education of young school students with severe speech, language and communication difficulties, it does not sit comfortably with traditional medical/therapy models of individual assessment.

Funding for communication aid technology

Funding (or lack of it) for the purchase of AAC technology and for the funding of appropriate ongoing specialist assessment and support services is often a major barrier to the effective use of AAC in schools, in many countries across the world. Sometimes, as in the UK currently, funding may be made available to accompany government initiatives for special educational needs students, but fails to be distributed equitably due to an absence of statutory entitlement to provision of AAC equipment and services, a lack of clear guidelines establishing which agencies are responsible for AAC provision to children, and persistent dislocation in practice, at national and local levels, between education, health and social services.

Particular funding difficulties may also be caused by the issues raised in the previous section, where the young child going through school is likely to require a sequence (and sometimes a simultaneous collection) of different AAC systems, over a period, rather than a 'one-off' purchase of a single system.

Quite apart from communication aid technology, it is important to remember that a budget is needed also for the non-trivial ongoing costs of low-tech AAC materials. Funding may also be required for appropriate seating, furniture, mounting systems(s) and peripherals— an AAC device is no use unless the child can access it effectively in the classroom and moving around the school.

The current trend towards use of standard hardware (*e.g.* the personal computer) rather than highly specialized 'black box technology' as the basis of AAC systems can be helpful in the school setting. If the child starts with use of an ordinary desktop computer running, for example, dynamic screen communication aid software, school staff may become comfortable with it, system use can be fully evaluated, and the child's progress and success with the system can be demonstrated and documented to support a funding request for a more expensive portable dedicated communication aid.

The curriculum and individual educational plans

Educating and supporting children with special educational needs involves trying to balance up the objectives of the national educational curriculum with the highly focused goals and targets of a student's own individual educational plan/programme (IEP). For AAC users, good collaborative practice between teachers and speech and language therapists should ensure that AAC competencies are integrated into the IEP.

NATIONAL CURRICULUM

In most countries, the national curriculum[1] is designed to provide a shared framework in all schools—mainstream and special—emphasizing breadth, balance and progression. It is expected that students with special educational needs will access the same curriculum as their peers, although different students will move through the stages of the curriculum at different rates. Teachers differentiate when they plan lessons and deliver the curriculum, recognizing that although students may be working on the same subject area, different teaching methods and approaches, and adjustment of attainment targets may be required to ensure appropriate learning experiences for every student. Special schools/units/classes may teach a version of the national curriculum that is more radically adapted, but should still be working within the overall framework. [A totally personalized curriculum, as Beukelman and Mirenda (1998) point out, risks isolating the student from peers, making them dependent on the philosophies of individual staff, and lowering expectations of students, staff and parents.] Although 'Language' is a specific curricular area in its own right, teaching and learning to use AAC should not be consigned to that area only as a learning objective, but incorporated across all curricular areas as a method of teaching and learning.

INDIVIDUAL EDUCATIONAL PLAN

An IEP is both a process and a formal document (in the USA, it has legal status), which performs the following functions (Tod *et al.* 1998):
* assessing/identifying the child's needs
* deciding how the school intends to meet those needs
* planning for progression—and setting out a timescale
* harnessing resources and using these appropriately and effectively
* coordinating the activity of teachers and special needs assistants
* providing a tool for monitoring the effectiveness of teaching and learning
* providing evidence for outside bodies (*e.g.* in the UK, OFSTED/HMI)
* identifying staff development needs.

Effective IEPs will (amongst other things):
* include input from parents and from the child, if possible
* be manageable
* include both long and short term aims
* identify clear and relevant SMART[2] targets (DfEE 1994, HMI Audit Unit 1999)

---

[1]In the UK: the National Curriculum (England and Wales); 5–14 Curriculum Guidelines (Scotland).
[2]SMART = specific, measurable, achievable, relevant, timed.

- define performance/success criteria, indicating when targets have been achieved
- trigger action plans that outline clear roles and responsibilities for all concerned.

The IEP therefore is a child's 'map' designed to lead to appropriate academic experience and achievement; it is essential that AAC is ensconced at the core of it, not 'tacked on' somewhere on the edge as an afterthought. The child's ability to use AAC to communicate effectively is not in itself the educational objective, but the means to access learning experiences, to acquire specific knowledge, and to participate in activities (Cottier *et al.* 1997).

Identifying appropriate targets and performance criteria and integrating these within curricular areas lies at the heart of good practice in the support of school students using AAC. Useful sources for specific ideas might be the Preschool AAC Checklist (Henderson 1992) and the Core AAC Curriculum (Robertson *et al.* 1996).

There are many difficulties here. As Cooper (1996) points out, IEP targets embody a behavioural approach to teaching, whereas communication—not least because it is a social- and context-linked behaviour—is an aspect of children's development that does not always lend itself to being broken down into small, measurable sub-tasks. Furthermore, IEP targets are generally exclusively student-focused, and do not include information about support needs.

For this reason, schools may find it helpful to draw up specific Action Plans (Glennen and deCoste 1997) that outline the AAC support tasks needed (and identify the relevant timescales and the people responsible for carrying out each of these). For example, Figure 6.1 shows items that might be included in an Action Plan covering a child's transition from the special needs base into specific mainstream classes.

This is more paperwork, which everybody hates, but the simple fact is that unless AAC targets are included specifically within educational IEPs and Action Plans, they will be 'invisible' to school staff, there will be no time in the school day for them, and the necessary work to achieve them will simply not be carried out.

IMPLEMENTING IEPS AND ACTION PLANS
Successfully implementing plans that integrate both educational and AAC targets demands imagination and a willingness to innovate. Classrooms are not always communicative environments, so may need to be specially redesigned or 'engineered' (Goossens *et al.* 1992, Burkhardt 1993, Goossens 1999) to support the development of communication skills.

Creating a communicative classroom
Key approaches are likely to include:
- creating accessible materials
- vocabulary selection and organization
- creating communication opportunities
- using communication in natural contexts
- using Aided Language Stimulation (ALS)/System for Augmenting Language (SAL)
- training communication partners.

117

Student: Fred Green Transition from special needs base to three mainstream class sessions Team members: Elizabeth White, SEN teacher; Mary Black, SNA; Robert Brown, speech and language therapist; Susan Gray, mainstream class teacher; John Gold, mainstream class SNA		
Timescale	*Action*	*Staff responsible*
June–August 2000	Identify vocabulary needs for use in Morning Circle Time, Music, Environmental Studies project session (Term I—Water, Term II—People Who Work for Us)	Susan Gray, Elizabeth White, John Gold
August 2000	Create symbol pages and voice output communication aid (VOCA) overlays with this new vocabulary	Mary Black
August 2000	Programme VOCA	Mary Black
August–September 2000	Develop at least three 'engineered' classroom activities for Fred to use this symbol vocabulary interactively	Robert Brown
August–September 2000	Demonstrate, and train mainstream classroom staff in how to prompt and support these activities (aided language stimulation)	Robert Brown, Susan Gray, Elizabeth White, John Gold

Fig. 6.1. Example of an Action Plan drawn up to cover child's transition from special needs to mainstream education classes.

Creating materials

Where students are using symbols as a means of language/meaning representation, they need relevant symbols to accompany curriculum-based work and project topics (as well as their own personal communication vocabulary). The key is advance planning. If projects and topics are established at least a term in advance, then the teacher and therapist can plan vocabulary and materials in good time to allow the classroom assistant to produce the corresponding symbol charts and work sheets. The 'means of production' (*i.e.* computer, symbol software and printer) must be in school, not in a distant therapy base. The system also has to ensure that the person making materials has time allocated for this task (which can be highly time-consuming).

Vocabulary selection, organization and updating

An important part of teaching and supporting a student's AAC programme lies in ensuring that the available vocabulary is appropriate. To be effective, vocabulary needs to match the user's age, gender, cultural background, and cognitive and linguistic skills. It should also be personalized, reflecting each individual's style and interests. Users' own wishes should be accommodated, and vocabulary will need to be reviewed and updated regularly. In school, vocabulary needs to include curriculum-linked language, not just personal communication vocabulary.

Vocabulary is often broken down into:

- *core vocabulary* (frequently used items, including social phrases and personal vocabulary, and a bank of single words used for basic sentence building)
- *fringe vocabulary* (including situation-based vocabulary, often organized by topic, *e.g.* swimming, choosing food, etc.).

Latham and Miles (2000) report that inappropriate vocabulary selection can be a major stumbling block to successful use of AAC devices in the classroom. Children often either have a vocabulary that is too limited/limiting or else are overloaded with vocabulary with no opportunity to learn any of it well. Adults controlling children's vocabulary selection tend to focus on what users might want to talk about (*i.e. fringe vocabulary*, curriculum/topic based). The vocabulary offered does not always relate to users' communicative or developmental needs. The Redway School communication framework (Latham and Miles 2001) shows how appropriate *core vocabulary* can be identified for children at different developmental levels of communicative and cognitive function. Lesson plans across the curriculum, differentiated appropriately for each child, can then set objectives based on language and communication functions, so that each child has access to the necessary vocabulary to achieve at their level.

PRE-STORED VOCABULARIES FOR COMMUNICATION AIDS

It may take too long for teachers or therapists to build up a personalized vocabulary from scratch for each child. Additionally, there may be a good argument for several students in a group to share much of the same vocabulary, to facilitate the organization of teaching and learning activities, and to support participation and interaction. In this situation, use of a pre-programmed vocabulary may be indicated, such as Ingfield Dynamic Vocabularies (Connor and Larcher 1997) or CALLtalk (Millar 2000), with additional personalization, for each student.

CONSULTING THE AAC USER, REVIEWING AND UPDATING VOCABULARY

Various techniques may help to ensure that the user's own priorities are included in the vocabulary selected and that the selection has validity in relation to the user's 'real life' in school and elsewhere. For example:

- brainstorming with the user and communication partners (school staff, classmates, family, friends) to identify gaps, and weed out irrelevant vocabulary, in the existing system
- completing a communication diary ('shadowing' the user through a typical day/week) and noting all communication needs in different situations, noting any communication breakdowns, strategies used (over a longer period of time)
- reviewing existing word lists (*e.g.* lists from natural speakers, pre-stored AAC vocabularies), marking any useful vocabulary ideas).

Regular vocabulary review dates should be included in planning for AAC users, and should probably be formally set, otherwise this may 'drift' for too long.

CREATING COMMUNICATION OPPORTUNITIES

To avoid passivity or students who can only respond but not initiate, specific opportunities

for active communication and participation need to be identified from the earliest stage. At the very least, one communication act per activity throughout the school day should be expected. The situation may need to be engineered and 'scripted' to ensure that it 'works' properly. Examples might include:
- making the student responsible for reporting a news item at 'Circle Time'
- 'sabotaging' classroom routines so that a student has to ask a question (*e.g.* to find belongings or claim a turn)
- providing a menu in advance so the student is prepared to order her/his own lunch in the dinner hall
- sending the student with a message or request to another member of school staff
- carrying out a simple questionnaire-based 'survey' of other students on a specific topic.

TEACHING AND USING COMMUNICATION IN NATURAL CONTEXTS
Johnson *et al.* (1996) stress that all teaching and practice of AAC use should be set in 'natural' contexts:

> "Scheduling a time interval in which to "teach language, communication, or social skills" is justified only when this instruction is in addition to that already provided within naturally occurring routines and interactions with peers without disabilities. It is sometimes necessary and desirable to practice skills that are difficult to perform or to role-play interactions in order to become more proficient. These interactions, along with other instructional practices, can enhance communication but must be coordinated within a systematic instructional plan of teaching during routines embedded in natural environments."

In other words, all activities and tasks should be as 'real' as possible, and should be:
- functional/meaningful/relevant in everyday situations, if possible
- motivating/fun in social and play situations, if possible
- interactive and sociable in dialogue and small group situations, if possible.

In the school setting, 'natural environments' would include classroom and playground interactions between peers and the ordinary day-to-day delivery of the curriculum in the classroom, in group settings. (It would not include the withdrawal of individual children for one-to one therapy.[1])

Goossens (1999) warns that many AAC group activities in special classes can look suspiciously like *"multiple one-on-one activities rather than true group activities"* that risk being boring and in which children are often simply waiting their turn (possibly for periods longer than their attention span).

USING AIDED LANGUAGE STIMULATION (ALS)/SYSTEM FOR AUGMENTING LANGUAGE (SAL)
These specialized approaches warrant more space than can be afforded to them in this

---

[1]Evidence collected from young people who are learning to use AAC indicates strongly that there is a need also for one-to-one therapy (Clarke *et al.* 2001b).

chapter. Basically, both are different types of 'immersion' techniques for providing students with a model to follow, in combining and using symbols, and for cueing students in to use symbols appropriately, in naturalistic situations.

TRAINING COMMUNICATION PARTNERS

Schools are notorious for a heavily directive style of communication—mainly teacher-led questioning. Training may need to be introduced for adults in the classroom to sensitize them to the need for more open-ended and linguistically diverse styles of communication, including conversational interaction, in order to provide balanced language use for the AAC user. Other children, involved as a part of peer tutor and 'buddy' systems for literacy (or other) instruction programmes, may also benefit from training programmes.

AAC and literacy

Things often go well in an inclusive setting for AAC users for the first three years of primary education when most work is oral, but may start to fall apart at the point where most teaching and recording of work is done through the medium of written language.

The issue in classrooms is often how to achieve the right balance between speaking/ listening/reading and writing. It has been known for AAC systems to be misused in schools, neglecting functional communication and conversation in favour of highly limited and limiting structured reading/writing tasks. Equally, it has been known for literacy instruction to be ignored or omitted, through a lack of understanding about how to tackle this, with non-speaking students.

It is well known that children with severe communication difficulties are likely to also experience difficulties with the acquisition of literacy, although there is plenty of evidence, too (Yoder and Koppenhaver 1993) that AAC users can be expected to acquire some degree of literacy, given exposure and adequate amounts of appropriate instruction. AAC users are likely to need a computer-based supportive writing aid, as well as a personal communication aid, and it will be important for use of the two to be closely integrated in a planned way.

Conclusion

Supporting children using AAC in schools has been shown to be a complex and challenging scenario, relying to a large extent for a successful outcome on policy makers, and senior school management who are in the position to enable the necessary 'back-up' for teachers and therapists, in the form of planning, training, funding and time allocation for joint, collaborative planning and working.

REFERENCES

American Speech–Language–Hearing Association (1993) 'Guidelines for caseload size and speech-language service delivery in the schools.' *ASHA*, **35**, Suppl. 10, 33–39.

Beukelman, D.R., Mirenda, P. (1998) *Augmentative and Alternative Communication: Management of Severe Communication Disorders in Children and Adults. 2nd Edn.* Baltimore: Paul H. Brookes.

Blackstone, S. (1995) 'AAC teams.' *Augmentative Communication News*, **8** (4), 1–3.

Blamires, M. (1999) 'What is enabling technology?' *In:* Blamires, M. (Ed.) *Enabling Technology for Inclusion.* London: Paul Chapman, pp. 1–16.

Burkhart, L. (1993) *Total Augmentative Communication in the Early Childhood Classroom.* Solana Beach, CA: Mayer Johnson.

Calculator, S.N, Jorgensen, C.M. (1991) 'Integrating AAC instruction into regular education settings: Expounding on best practices.' *Augmentative and Alternative Communication*, 7, 204–214.

Chinnery, S., Hazell, G., Skinner, P., Thomas, P., Williams, G. (2001) *Developing Augmentative and Alternative Communication Policies in Schools.* Headington, Oxford: ACE Centre Advisory Trust.

Clarke, M., McConachie, H., Price, K., Wood, P. (2001a) 'Speech and language therapy provision for children using augmentative and alternative communication systems.' *European Journal of Special Needs Education*, 16, 41–54.

—— —— —— —— (2001b) 'Views of young people using augmentative and alternative communication systems.' *International Journal of Language and Communication Disorders*, 36, 107–115.

Connor, S., Larcher, J. (1997) 'Development of Ingfield Vocabularies.' *Communication Matters*, 11 (3), 5–7.

Cooper, P. (1996) 'Are Individual Education Plans a waste of paper?' *British Journal of Special Education*, 23, 115–119.

Cottier, C., Doyle, M., Gilworth, K. (1997) *Functional AAC Intervention: A Team Approach.* Winslow, Oxfordshire: Imaginart.

Cunningham, C., Davies, H. (1985) *Working with Parents: Frameworks for Collaboration.* Milton Keynes: OUP.

Department for Education and Employment (DfEE) (1994) *Code of Practice on the Identification and Assessment of Special Educational Needs.* Sudbury, Suffolk: DfEE Publications.

Donnelly, J. (2000) 'Introducing symbols to special education.' *In:* Wilson, A. (Ed.) *AAC 2000. Practical Approaches to Augmentative and Alternative Communication.* Edinburgh: CALL Centre, University of Edinburgh, pp. 36–41.

Downing, J. (1999) *Teaching Communication Skills to Students with Severe Disabilities.* Baltimore: Paul Brookes.

Farmer, H., Reid, J. (2001) *How Good Iis Our Collaboration? Working Practice Agreements Between Schools and Speech and Language Therapists.* Cardenden, Fife: Fife Council Education Service.

Glennen, S.L., DeCoste, D.C. (1997) *The Handbook of Augmentative and Alternative Communication.* San Diego: Singular Publishing.

Goossens, C. (1999) *Creating a Communicative Classroom. Proceedings of the AAC Study Days, Dunfermline and Lancaster, 17 and 29 September 1999.*

—— Crain, S.S., Elder, P.S. (1992) *Engineering the Preschool Environment for Interactive Symbolic Communication.* Birmingham, AL: Southeast Augmentative Communication Conference Publications.

Grove, N., Norwich, B. (1997) *Children Using Augmentative and Alternative Communication in London Schools: Estimates of Prevalence and Profiles of Use.* Research report presented tothe Mercers Company & Micro Assistance in Continuing Education, Institute of Education, University of London.

Henderson, J. (1992) *Preschool AAC Checklist.* Solana Beach, CA: Mayer-Johnson.

HMI Audit Unit (1999) *Raising Standards—Setting Targets for Pupils with Special Educational Needs.* Edinburgh: Scottish Office Education & Industry Department.

ICAC (1995) *Communication Aids for Children: Guidelines to Good Practice.* London: AFASIC.

Johnson, J.M., Baumgart, D., Helmstetter, E., Curry, C.A. (1996) *Augmenting Basic Communication in Natural Contexts.* Baltimore: Paul H. Brookes.

Kersner, M., Wright, J. (1996) 'Collaboration between teachers and speech and language therapists working with children with severe learning difficulties (SLD): implications for professional development.' *British Journal of Learning Disabilities*, 24, 33–37.

Koppenhaver, D.A., Steelman, J.D., Pierce, P.L., Yoder, D., Staples, A. (1993) 'Developing augmentative and alternative communication technology in order to develop literacy.' *Technology and Disability*, 2 (3), 32–42.

Kraat, A. (1985) *Communication Interaction Between Aided and Natural Speakers: A State of the Art Report.* Toronto: Canadian Rehabilitation Council for the Disabled.

Lacey, P., Lomas, L. (1993) *Support Services and the Curriculum: a Practical Guide to Collaboration.* London: David Fulton.

Latham, C., Miles. A. (2000) 'Making the curriculum work for VOCAs: the Redway School model.' *Communication Matters*, 14 (2), 10–12.

—— —— (2001) *Communication and the Curriculum.* London: David Fulton.

Light, J. (1989) 'Towards a definition of communicative competence for individuals using augmentative and alternative communication systems.' *Augmentative and Alternative Communication*, 5, 137–144.

122

Martin, D., Miller, C. (1999) *Language and the Curriculum: Practitioner Research in Planning Differentiation.* London: David Fulton.

McConachie, H., Pennington, L. (1997) 'In-service training for schools on augmentative and alternative communication.' *European Journal of Disorders of Communication,* **32,** 277–288.

Mendes, E., Rato, J. (1996) 'From system to communication: staff training for attitude change.' *In:* von Tetzchener, S., Jensen M. (Eds.) *European Perspectives on Augmentative and Alternative Communication.* London: Whurr, pp. 342–354.

Millar, S. (1998) 'The child, education, and augmentative and alternative communication.' *In:* Wilson, A. (Ed.) *Augmentative Communication in Practice: An Introduction.* Edinburgh: CALL Centre, University of Edinburgh, pp. 54–61.

—— (2001) 'CALLtalk: a new dynamic screen communication vocabulary.' *In:* Wilson, A. (Ed.) *AAC 2000. Practical Approaches to Augmentative and Alternative Communication.* Edinburgh: CALL Centre, University of Edinburgh, pp. 58–62.

—— Larcher, J., Robinson, P. (1999) 'Dynamic screen communication systems.' *Communication Matters,* **13** (3), 27–31.

Murphy, J. Markova, I., Moodie, E., Scott, J., Boa, S. (1995) 'Augmentative and alternative communication systems used by people with cerebral palsy in Scotland: demographic survey.' *Augmentative and Alternative Communication,* **11,** 26–30.

——Collins, S., Moodie, E. (1996) 'AAC Systems: obstacles to effective use.' *European Journal of Disorders of Communication,* **31,** 31–44.

Office of Special Education Programs (OSEP) (2000) *22nd Annual Report to Congress on the Implementation of the Individuals with Disabilities Education Act.* Washington DC: US Department of Education.

Pennington, L., Jolleff, N., McConachie, H., Wisbeach, A., Price, K. (1993) *My Turn to Speak: A Team Approach to Augmentative Communication.* London: Institute of Child Health.

Phillips, B., Zhao, H. (1993) 'Predictors of assistive technology abandonment.' *Assistive Technology,* **5,** 36–45.

Pickles, P.A.C. (1998) *Managing the Curriculum for Children with Severe Motor Difficulties: A Practical Approach.* London: David Fulton.

Reid, J., Farmer, H. (2000) *How Good Is Our Collaboration?* Fife Education Department, ASDARC, Cardenden, Fife.

—— Millar, S., Tait, L., Donaldson, M. Dean, E., Thomson, G.O.B., Grieve, R. (1996) *The Role of Speech and Language Therapists in the Education of Pupils with Special Educational Needs.* Edinburgh: Centre for Research in Child Development.

Robertson. J., and the CORE team (1996) *The Core AAC Curriculum.* London: SCOPE.

Romski, M.A., Sevcik, R.A. (1992) 'Developing augmented language in children with severe mental retardation.' *In:* Warren, S.F., Reichle, J. (Eds.) *Communication and Language Intervention Series: Vol. 2. Enhancing Children's Communication.* Baltimore: Paul Brookes, pp. 85–104.

Royal College of Speech and Language Therapists (RCSLT) (1996) *Communicating Quality 2: Professional Standards for Speech and Language Therapists.* London: RCSLT.

Scottish Office Education and Industry Department (SOEID) (1996) *The Education of Pupils with Language and Communication Disorders: A Report by HM Inspectors of Schools.* Edinburgh: The Scottish Office.

—— (1999) *A Manual of Good Practice in Special Educational Needs: Professional Practice in Meeting SEN.* Edinburgh: The Scottish Office.

Soto, G. (1997) 'Special education teacher attitudes towards AAC: Preliminary survey.' *Augmentative and Alternative Communication,* **13,** 186–196.

Thomson, G.O.B., Stewart, M.E., Ward, K. (1995) *Criteria for Opening Records of Needs.* Edinburgh: SOED.

Tod, J., Castle, F., Blamires, M. (1998) *IEPs—Implementing Effective Practice.* London: David Fulton.

United Nations (1993) *Standard Rules on the Equalization of Opportunities for Persons with Disabilities. 85th Plenary Meeting, 20 December 1993. A/RES/48/96.*

United Nations Educational, Scientific and Cultural Organization (UNESCO) (1994) *The Salamanca Statement and Framework for Action on Principles, Policy and Practice in Special Education. ED-94/WS/18.*

Wright, J. (1996) 'Teachers and therapists: the evolution of a partnership.' *Child Language Teaching and Therapy,* **12,** 3–16.

Wylie, C. (2000) *Picking up the Pieces: Review of Special Education 2000.* New Zealand Research Council (url: www.executive.govt.nz/minister/dalziel/index.html).

Yoder, D., Koppenhaver, D. (1993) 'Classroom literacy instruction for children with severe speech and physical impairments (SSPI): What is and what might be.' *Topics in Language Disorder,* **13** (2), 1–15.

7

THE IMPACT OF ADOLESCENCE ON THE USE OF VOICE OUTPUT COMMUNICATION AIDS

Pam Stevenson

This chapter examines the factors that influence the attitude of the adolescent with unintelligible speech to voice output communication equipment. The responses of the young person at this time will often be unpredictable and difficult to understand, not least by the user her/himself.

Adolescence is characterized by a broadening of horizons with increased social activity (Thomas *et al.* 1989), the growing importance of the peer group, fluctuations in mood and behaviour (Coleman and Hendry 1991), awareness, and often criticism of, bodily changes (Davies and Furnham 1986) and the emergence of sexuality (West 1999).

Studies of adolescents with chronic disabilities, including cerebral palsy, demonstrate their vulnerability. The group of young people with spina bifida studied by Castree and Walker (1981) were characterized by increasing social isolation. Pless and Stein (1994) reviewed the research into the risk that chronic disorders confer for maladjustment. All the findings confirmed "the presence of significant risk for various kinds of emotional disturbance in the presence of a chronic illness". In their sample of 286 young adults with chronic health conditions, Ireys *et al.* (1994) identified the presence of speech and hearing problems as one of the conditions heightening the risk of poor mental health.

Many studies show an increased incidence of divorce in families with a disabled child (Mauldon 1992). A number of studies, *e.g.* Walczac and Burns (1984), have described the strong and painful emotions, including distress, rejection, anger and unhappiness, experienced by the child following family breakdown. Coleman and Hendry (1991) stress the need for teenagers to have good communication with parents at this time. They review Wallerstein and Kelly's (1980) study, which showed a direct relationship between post-divorce adjustment and the degree of communication between them and their parents. They also showed that young people, particularly adolescents, were "clamouring for more information, and for the opportunity to be involved in decisions which they feel directly affect their lives". There are implications for the provision of appropriate AAC equipment,vocabulary and supportive training to help non-speaking teenagers deal with this need.

The young people discussed in this chapter are, or have recently been, students at Treloar School, Froyle, Hampshire, England, a non-maintained special school for children aged 5 to 16 years. Names have been changed in the case studies. The school has the advantage of being well resourced, both with specialist staff and with AAC equipment. The need for multidisciplinary assessment, when prescribing AAC equipment and monitoring its use, is recognized (Jolleff *et al.* 1992). To meet this need the school has a well-established Communication Support Team comprising speech and language therapists, an occupational therapist, a special needs teacher, a rehabilitation engineer and the AAC coordinator. The school is residential with some day places. There is an opportunity to study communication needs in a variety of situations, and to implement training for relevant teaching and care staff and for interested others, such as gardeners and porters. Regular contact with parents can be difficult, however. While the issues discussed here are relevant to adolescents growing up in any setting, it may be that residential schooling has both positive and negative impacts.

The need to fully involve parents in decisions about communication equipment is stressed by Granlund and colleagues (Chapter 5). Despite the growing importance of the peer group, parents are undoubtedly prominent figures who continue to influence the adolescent's life (Tatar 1998).

The following issues concerning the use of AAC by adolescents will be illustrated by case studies: protective factors for mental health; parental influence; parental separation; the need for personal vocabulary; coming to terms with disability; competence and self-esteem; body image; learning difficulties; sexual maturation; speed of AAC access; and poor physical health.

Protective factors for mental health and parental influence
CASE STUDY
Alex Brown transferred to Treloar School aged 14. He had cerebral palsy with spastic quadriplegia and with no intelligible speech. He was a thoughtful boy whose behaviour in his first year showed considerable anxiety. He frequently asked staff to phone his father to let him know of some change or to ask permission about various, apparently trivial, things. He lived with his father in the holidays; his mother had moved away and remarried. Staff contact with Alex's father was not easy; he lived hundreds of miles away and ran a business that made it difficult for him to leave home, and Alex was collected and delivered to school by taxis at the beginning and end of school holidays.

When Alex arrived at Treloar School, he communicated with a large word board, comprising core and fringe vocabulary, which he used effectively to build up grammatical sentences by pointing to the words with his thumb. This board was hung from the back of his wheelchair. He also had a Cameleon (modified personal computer) mounted on his chair, accessed by a touch screen with 'Talking Screen' software. He was using a 'speech set' that had been largely developed by his father. Talking Screen is a symbol-based programme that allows the user to move between topic 'pages' to assemble, and then speak, messages. In his first term, Alex made efforts to use this but often resorted to asking for his word board. Examination of his programme revealed that, although there were a large number of pre-stored sentences to enable Alex to talk effectively about his family or his passion for football, vocabulary was organized in such a way that generating grammatical novel utterances was far more difficult. Alex's use of his word board had demonstrated his intact inner language, and he was demonstrating his lively intelligence in all areas of the school. It became apparent that Talking Screen, even with extensive re-programming, would not meet his needs in his current situation.

The Communication Support Team looked at other options, and EZ Keys (a literacy-based programme that would give Alex a far more flexible communication tool), was loaded into the Cameleon, alongside Talking Screen, and used in English lessons. Alex was demonstrating considerable difficulty with spelling and an inability to guess at initial letters of new words. Further assessments revealed severe phonological processing difficulties, which ruled out the use of EZ Keys for communication.

It was decided to look at 'semantic compaction', the system used in Liberator voice output communication equipment where a fixed overlay of icons (multi-meaning pictures) is used to generate hundreds of words and phrases. The user can access the stored messages using a logical system of combinations of icons, known as 'Minspeak'. This system is akin to learning a foreign language, and it was with some trepidation that this course was embarked upon, because Alex had now less than two years ahead of him at Treloar School.

The need to change software, and possibly hardware, was broached with Alex's father in phone calls. Understandably, he was not enthusiastic, having learned how to programme the Cameleon and spent hours building up a personalized programme for his son. Although he gave the Treloar speech and language therapist the go-ahead to work with Liberator equipment with Alex, it was not clear he was convinced that the change was necessary. Alex began using the Liberator, with a powerful Minspeak Application Programme (MAP), called 'Language Learning and Living' in individual speech and language therapy sessions. In these he was making progress and he was included in a small group of students using the same programme. At the February half-term break and at Easter he took the Liberator home with him (as well as his Cameleon) to show his father. Each time, he returned without having used it. Vocabulary that had been learned had been forgotten. He remained keen to use the Liberator in school, but was clearly very concerned not to upset his father.

The speech and language therapist had further phone conversations with Alex's father, explaining about Alex's intelligence, inner language, spelling difficulties, etc. In July, Mr Brown attended Alex's annual educational review at which Alex was present. Again the issues surrounding Alex's communication equipment were aired, together with reports of his patchy progress with the Liberator. At the end of the review Mr Brown announced, "I think the Liberator is now the best communication equipment for Alex, and I think he's just been waiting to hear me say so." From that day Alex made exponential progress. He returned after the Summer holidays speaking in long grammatical sentences, having absorbed the logic of the programme, built on the vocabulary he had been taught, and independently explored and learned new vocabulary.

Alex's final year was characterized by a marked reduction in anxiety. He was now able to express his strong sense of humour and to take an active part in group discussions. He did well in a number of certificated courses and moved on to Treloar College where, amongst other things, he gained a recognized qualification in AAC. He continues to be an expert Liberator user and was recently made a Platinum level Ambassador by the distributors, to represent them at meetings, conferences, etc.

Alex had been at risk of becoming chronically anxious. The improvement in his ability to communicate and express his concerns appeared to help prevent this, despite the presence of other risk factors such as marital breakdown. The need for Alex to have his father's unequivocal 'permission' to change his communication equipment highlights the need for good parent/professional relationships.

Parental separation

As mentioned above, communication is particularly important for adolescents who are living through the process of family breakdown. They will need vocabulary that will enable them to talk about their reactions.

CASE STUDY

Ryan had cerebral palsy with moderate learning difficulties, a long history of disturbed behaviour, and some autistic features. From the age of 12 years his behaviour gradually began to improve, and his obsessional and autistic traits diminished. During this time he communicated with some, very dysarthric, speech and with his symbol-based word book. At the age of 15 he began showing interest in using high-tech communication equipment, for the first time. Not fully literate, he was provided with a DeltaTalker, on which a custom-made programme was developed, using the Minspeak logic described above. The DeltaTalker is similar to the Liberator; it is slimmer and lighter but has a reduced number of features.

While he was in the early stages of learning to use this, his parents separated. Confused and upset, he went between members of staff seeking explanations with the words, "Why Mum Dad no love?" On another occasion he was able to express his fears that he would lose contact with his father; he groaned "Oh no" (with his voice) and then said "Goodbye Dad" with his DeltaTalker. He has subsequently gone on to accept the situation, in part due to his ability to explain his concerns.

Private vocabulary

There is also a need for non-speaking, non-literate adolescents to have access to vocabulary with which to discuss personal matters that may be concerning them, such as menstruation or the other physical changes that come with puberty. Many young people refuse to have such embarrassing vocabulary stored on their communication equipment in case it is spoken by mistake. Similarly, they rarely allow these topics to be added to their communication books. One way round this is to provide care staff with a private book of 'delicate' vocabulary and to teach the student its contents. There is also a need to provide young people with the sort of 'rude' vocabulary that they will hear from their peers. They will sometimes have to be taught where and when not to use this. There is something offensive about seeing, written down, strong vocabulary that would be acceptable if heard spoken in the right context. For example, a communication aid user may request the words "Push off!" (or worse) to be stored for use with someone who is annoying her/him. This can be stored in such a way that a startled passer-by, checking that s/he had heard correctly, would read, "Would you mind going away" on the screen.

Coming to terms with disability

Adolescence is the time when young people become more aware of their disability, and the restrictions that come with it. Coming to terms with the need for communication equipment can be enormously stressful, both for the adolescent and for parents who may have continued to hope that speech would improve as their child grew older. They may have received mixed prognoses from professionals, the progress of dyspraxic and dysarthric speech being very difficult to predict (Bodine and Beukerman 1991).

There is concern about the future, focused by the realization that adulthood approaches. In a study of able-bodied adolescents, Coleman *et al.* (1977) found that young people's fears and anxieties about themselves as they grew older appeared to be very much more common in those about to leave school.

Perhaps surprisingly, severity of disability is not related in a simple manner to the extent of psychological difficulties experienced by the adolescent. Studies, reviewed by Ireys *et al.* (1994), relating severity of illness to mental health, are inconclusive, partly due to a variable definition of severity (Stein *et al.* 1987). However, Jessop and Stein (1985) found that children with conditions that produce marginal impairment have more psychological problems than their severely disabled peers.

CASE STUDY

Claire transferred to Treloar School at the age of 14, with the request from her parents and her Local Education Authority that she be assessed and provided with communication equipment. She had suffered meningitis at the age of a few weeks, which had resulted in a very slight left hemiplegia. Her speech was severely affected; originally diagnosed as aphasic and dysarthric, the diagnosis was later changed to dyspraxia. An intelligent, attractive girl with good hand control and normal gait, there was no visible sign of her disability, unless she was asked to smile or stick out her tongue, both of which she could do involuntarily but not voluntarily. At interview, Claire was provided with a Lightwriter and used it effectively to type out messages, being literate, with good use of syntax and with normal hand control. The process of prescription was straightforward: the Lightwriter was the obvious choice, being small, discreet, easy to carry around with a shoulder strap, and easy to hold while typing. Dual display screens face both user and listener, and the Lightwriter has speech output.

Implementation was not so easy. Claire was initially happy that the equipment was to be bought for her, but her attitude was ambivalent. She had attended a school where the emphasis had been on traditional speech and language therapy, and she had attended daily sessions. Another change was the fact that her previous school had been a signing school, unlike Treloar School where too few of the students have sufficiently good hand control to make this method of communication viable.

It became clear that she believed if she practised enough, her speech would become intelligible. In fact, although she occasionally uttered single words or short phrases clearly, her connected speech was impossible to understand, even when reading from a text that her listener could see. Claire was very anxious to attend for articulation work and she was given two sessions per week, which included some exercises, even though it was apparent that the more Claire tried the more difficult accurate articulation became. These sessions were also used for discussion of communication generally, and during them she frequently became angry and impatient, saying, with her Lightwriter, that her previous speech and language therapist had understood her speech perfectly.

Claire had been gently persuaded by her form tutor to have her Lightwriter ready at hand for occasions when she was not understood in class, and teachers were aware of the sensitivity of the situation. She still preferred to use a tiny notebook and pencil, which she carried in her pocket, and continued to reject the Lightwriter. Key staff learnt some signs and finger spelling. Her speech and language therapist suggested seeking out signing conversation classes, to maintain her signing ability, but Claire chose not to do this. Instead she agreed to teach signing to a group of friends and care staff, and her speech and language therapist helped her to advertise and plan these sessions.

It was a very stressful time for Claire, coping with the demands of GCSEs, forging friendships in a new peer group and pressured by both her (separated) parents to use the Lightwriter, which they saw as important for her future. She refused formal counselling but chose to talk to one or two members of the school staff, and discussed issues surrounding her schoolwork or her disability at length. Her emotional turmoil manifested itself in short-lived tantrums followed by apologies.

In speech and language therapy sessions Claire began to talk about traumatic communication experiences. For example, she described her embarrassment when asked for her order in a café by a waiter, while she was briefly alone at a table. She began to take on the idea of total communication; that she used her voice, some signs and gesture, and her Lightwriter. French vocabulary, phonetically written, was stored into her Lightwiter, enabling her to gain an oral score and pass her GCSE French examination. However, as she explained some years later, it was the realization that it enabled her to join in peer group banter that finally led her to accept her AAC equipment. This process had taken two years. She reported that the Lightwriter had gone on to become "an inseparable friend". Claire moved on to Treloar College from where she attended a Sixth Form College. She passed higher level examinations and went to University.

At school, Claire's disabilities had been considerably less complex than those of most of her peers. It was this apparent normality that appeared to be a factor in her very stormy adolescence. There is little doubt that if communication equipment had been prescribed without the emotional support, it would have been rejected.

The effect of competence on self-esteem

The importance of self-esteem, in the maintenance of overall well-being in adolescence, is stressed by Rosenberg (1979). Various studies, including that of Harter (1983) conclude that competence, or success in meeting achievement demands, is one of the factors underlying self-esteem. Rosenberg stresses that it is the importance that an individual attaches to a particular activity that will affect self-esteem. He gives the example that the adolescent's lack of prowess in physical skills may not have a negative effect if s/he does not view these as important.

CASE STUDY
Matthew has cerebral palsy with spastic quadriplegia and no speech. An intelligent boy, at

the age of 12 he was fully literate and used a word book with colour coding to help access by eye pointing. The decision was made to provide him with a Cameleon running EZ Keys software.

Access was an issue that was less easy to resolve. Matthew was adamant that he would only use his hands, despite having very poor hand control particularly for fine movement. This meant that he was confined to scanning using a single switch. The switch was positioned centrally on his tray and access was both slow and effortful; it was also noisy and distracting for other members of the class. At this time Matthew was an angry young man. His awareness of his disability, and the resentment that he felt for the able bodied, were expressed in his written work. His devoted (single) mother did her best to support him. She reported that his father had been dismissive about his hand control, and it was for this reason that Matthew was very keen to prove everyone wrong. He persevered with the use of the switch and became adept at using it; however, his chosen method of access continued to be both slow and noisy. He quickly learned his way around the programme and how to use the on-screen mouse emulator to access other programmes. Occupational therapists and rehabilitation engineers carried out timed trials that showed Matthew that head switch use would be much quicker, but to no avail. At the same time Matthew refused to contemplate supportive seating, or to have a knee block or his feet strapped. This resulted in poor posture and a position that was far from ideal for hand function.

There were a number of early software problems with EZ Keys, affecting several Cameleon-using students. Newer versions of the programme removed the bugs but not before they had caused everyone considerable frustration. This was compounded by the fact that as personal computers, the Cameleons were being used for word processing in addition to communication. Other students' Cameleons began working normally, but not so Matthew's. His speech and language therapist continued to receive almost daily messages from school staff, and from Matthew's mother, reporting problems. EZ Keys crashed, Microsoft Word 'disappeared', core system files were lost, voice output changed and more. On some occasions Matthew was brought up to the speech and language therapy department with tears pouring down his cheeks. A phone call to the manufacturer resulted in apologies to Matthew, and the Cameleon was repeatedly sent back for repair. Some six months later, a new computer systems manager at Treloar School discovered that Matthew was systematically sabotaging the software; he had been doing this at times when no-one was watching, using his single switch. The computer specialist wrote a programme to lock him out of certain areas, and to hide a copy of Word so that it reloaded on next rebooting. It was realized that Matthew had found it very rewarding to bewilder staff, and so a 'no fuss' response to breakdowns was adopted. For a while Matthew continued to try to find ways of causing problems, but then gave up, perhaps realizing that he had, at last, met his match.

Matthew has matured. At the age of 16 he has agreed to moulded seating for his wheelchair, which has opened the way for a reassessment of access. He is having a trial with a head mouse, a wireless optical sensor that interacts with a small reflective dot worn on the forehead. Most importantly he is a happier young man, who now jokes about the time when he sabotaged his software. He uses his Cameleon constructively to communicate and to word process, plays an active part in communication groups, and works hard in class.

Matthew has worked through his adolescent anger, and it seems reasonable to assume that this process, and his self-esteem, were helped by his prowess with his Cameleon, plus his ability to discuss megabytes of RAM and gigabytes of hard drive, and not least by his ability to hoodwink staff. He has skills of which he is justifiably proud.

Conflict and the move towards independence

It is not easy for young people with total care needs to move from dependency towards independence from their parents. As in the able-bodied adolescent, the transition is almost certain to involve some conflict (Coleman and Hendry 1991). It is tempting to think that efficient communication is the key to this process and that it will be valued by everyone; occasionally young people deliver a salutary reminder that they have other priorities.

CASE STUDY

Laura joined the school at the age of 13. She had spastic quadriplegia with no use of her hands, and speech that was intelligible to those who were very familiar with her speech, within a limited context. She had been prescribed a Cameleon and her wheelchair had been equipped with an 8+8 interface to allow her to use an integrated system. An 8+8 is an electronic box that interfaces between a wheelchair, communication equipment and, if required, a computer or environmental controls. Using a set of head switches, Laura could scan and select one of eight wheelchair directional controls, or change modes to operate her communication equipment. She was using EZ Keys software for word processing and to support her speech, but she saw herself primarily as a speaker.

Laura's parents had been very keen that she should use her communication equipment, but in her teenage years she was beginning to reject the technology for which her parents had fought so hard. She consented to have it mounted on her wheelchair but refused to have it turned on, ready for use. This meant that if she needed to speak to someone who did not understand her, there was a delay of several minutes while the machine booted up. She used it well in class and in communication groups, but used speech with her friends. She was very proud of her stylish new wheelchair, was very clothes conscious, and seemed to be moving inexorably towards refusing to have the Cameleon on her chair. The rehabilitation engineers reduced the size of her head switches, to her specification, and her mother made leopardskin covers for them. Ultimately however, Laura asked for the Cameleon to be taken off her chair, much to her parents' dismay. She continued to use it on her desk in class for written work. Her speech and language therapist had to explain that, at the age of 16, Laura was entitled to make this decision.

She was, in many ways, a very normal teenager, very interested in fashion, her peer group and boys. She felt that she could get by using speech in most situations and was not concerned that teachers could not understand her. There may have been an element of rebellion against her parents' wishes. She left school with the skills to use her communication equipment effectively, in situations of her choice.

Body image

As Coleman and Hendry (1991) point out, "Being liked, accepted, and finding one's identity

in a group are important at any age, but may be particularly crucial during adolescence."
This need is focused on the way the young person thinks s/he appears to others. Girls care
intensely about their body image in their teens (Rosenberg 1979).

Nancy joined Treloar School at the age of 12 with a Liberator that she accessed with a wafer
switch; this is a flat pad with five circles acting as up, down, left, right, and fire, as in a joystick. She had spastic quadriplegia. An intelligent girl, she made steady progress with the
mastery of her communication programme (Language Learning and Living) and became
fluent in its use, with good use of syntax and the stored vocabulary. Nancy's literacy skills
were improving and she was able to spell words for which she could not remember the icon
sequence. Her use of the equipment socially was limited, and she rarely chose to use her
Liberator at home.

Nancy's use of the wafer switch was slow, and following switch trials, head switches
were chosen and her speed of access improved. An increase in use followed; however, within
months there were reports that the Liberator was again being rejected. Nancy began to
complain that the head switches gave her neck pain. This complaint was taken seriously,
because of the dangers of repetitive strain injury. After discussion with Nancy's physiotherapist
it was decided to use a small round (brightly coloured) switch called a Jelly Bean, attached
to the side of her wheelchair for her to access with her knee. She had considerably less spasm
in her legs than in her arms. This was a movement that Nancy could control easily, and she
was, initially, delighted. Again there was increased use of the Liberator, followed by a reduction. Nancy's speech and language therapist regularly talked to her about her attitude
to her communication equipment, to try to understand the root of her reluctance, as did her
occupational therapist, who at that time was taking her on outings for community skills training. Nancy clearly didn't really know what the problem was; she declined assessment on
other hardware and said she loved her Liberator. Finally she told her occupational therapist
(with her Liberator) that she felt not using her hands for access made her look more disabled.
She would like to directly access her Liberator with her hand. Nancy's physiotherapist,
occupational therapist and speech and language therapist worked together with Nancy to
try to achieve this. There was real concern that by crashing down on the Liberator, and using
her knuckle to activate the small keys, Nancy would damage her hand. Different input
settings and keyguards were tried and a leather glove was made for Nancy to protect her
knuckle. No-one was convinced that Nancy would be able to reliably access like this, but
her motivation had soared. She persevered and at last seemed happy with her access method.
For Nancy the loss of communication efficiency was outweighed by other priorities.

Nancy was another student for whom communication was not of paramount importance.
She was interested in music, clothes and sport, and was an expert Boccia player. Nancy's
wish to normalize, as far as possible, her use of her communication equipment, was a need
that took a long time for her to understand and to express.

Learning difficulties

For children with significant learning difficulties, adolescence is likely to have a different impact. The family often remains central to their lives, with the peer group appearing to be of less importance. Other adolescent changes do occur, in line with the physical changes of puberty; there is increased interest in the opposite sex, and girls become interested in babies. Pop groups, clothes and make-up are important, but there is usually a passive enjoyment of these things, rather than an active involvement. The need to encourage young people to make choices and to initiate communication becomes increasingly relevant in adolescence, as they move towards adulthood. It is the time when parents and carers become aware of the need for a measure of independence.

Non-speaking children often develop a nonverbal system of communication with the family, which excludes outsiders. Parents become very skilled in interpreting their child's signals. Ko *et al.* (1998), analysing questionnaires completed by the parents of 30 children, found no evidence that parents perceived a marked change in children's communicative behaviour resulting from the use of augmentative communication systems. If a young person is only interested in communicating with close family, and that family does not find voice output equipment helps communication, it will be hard to engender motivation and enthusiasm for the task of mastering it. This can be the case even where parents support its use and collaborate in the choice of vocabulary.

In some instances the lack of communication equipment can be a focus of parental anguish; parents see others using voice output aids and feel that there must be a way for their child to benefit from technology. Sadly it is the case that if a young person has no ability or will to communicate with low-tech methods, using photos, pictures or symbols, or 'medium-tech' ones with one-hit spoken messages, high-tech methods may be of no, or very limited, help. This is particularly true when access to the equipment has to be by scanning with switches; the cognitive load may be too great.

When prescribing or upgrading voice output equipment it is important to look at language abilities. The level of language comprehension is crucial; it is appropriate to provide high-tech equipment where there is a significant discrepancy between comprehension and the young person's ability to express her/himself. A user may have a specific problem with expressive language affecting syntax and the ability to generate grammatical sentences, known as inner language, which might not become apparent until s/he is using voice output equipment if s/he is non-literate. This will cause problems of intelligibility; it is always easier to understand speech, especially synthetic speech, if it is grammatical. It need not be a counter-indicator to the provision of equipment if comprehension and the will to communicate are there. The user may need to rely more on stored phrases and sentences; listeners will have to put more work into interpreting messages. This can be combined with basic language work on word order.

Passivity is one of the greatest hurdles to progress with communication; it is perhaps a form of withdrawal or 'avoidant coping', described by Seiffge-Krenke (2000) as a coping mechanism in response to stress. One Treloar day student with moderate learning difficulties, visual problems and poor hand function was passive and not motivated to use her word book to speak to others; she gave ambiguous yes/no responses, and was not interested in trials with high-tech communication equipment. A symbol with the words "I have an appointment" was put in her word book. She began asking people to push her to the Medical

Centre several times a day for nonexistent appointments, to her obvious enjoyment, and to the delight of her speech and language therapist. This mischief-making has been part of a slow steady improvement in her participation at school, opening the way to the use of voice output equipment.

Multiple reasons for restricted use

A variety of factors can simultaneously affect the adolescent's use of her/his communication equipment. One apparent problem can mask others. In the following case study, AAC equipment is not being fully used for three separately identifiable reasons: sexual maturation, slow speed of access, and poor physical health.

CASE STUDY

Peter joined Treloar school at the age of 11, using Talking Screen, the symbol-based programme described above, on a Cameleon. He has cerebral palsy with athetosis, affecting all four limbs. His access was via a wafer switch. He was a lively boy with age-appropriate comprehension and great motivation to communicate. He had already begun to find 'Talking Screen' too restricting and frequently selected the spelling page with which to spell out words not stored. It was decided to move him on to EZ Keys, a literacy-based programme; he worked hard and mastered the programme quickly. Peter decided to continue with EZ Keys, for a while using the less demanding 'Talking Screen' programme in the evenings. Spelling was not a strong point, but with intensive literacy help he made considerable improvement. Peter expressed a wish to use a joystick to access his Cameleon, and with a new wheelchair and improved seating this became possible. However, communication was always going to be slow, physically effortful and cognitively demanding for him.

At the age of 15 Peter had become very interested in girls. Clearly the presence of a computer in front of you restricts your freedom to put your arm round your girlfriend, and Peter began choosing to have his Cameleon stowed behind his wheelchair on a foldaway mounting system. The rehabilitation engineers made screen protectors to prevent damage to the Cameleon when it was being carried in this position. Peter was adept at using facial expression, eye pointing and a few vocalizations to get his message across.

He continued to use his communication equipment effectively, but expressed the wish to try some faster method of communication. Speed is difficult to achieve, particularly using scanning. Instead of directly touching, or selecting with an infra-red beam, the user activates a switch or switches to direct or interrupt a sequentially highlighted display. A joystick moves the highlighted area to the location of the user's choice. No-one expects a wheelchair to be able to go up stairs, but people are sometimes unrealistic about the speed of communication that is possible when using voice output devices. This may be, in some part, the fault of the media, who broadcast interviews with the Cambridge astrophysicist Stephen Hawking without explaining either that they have edited out long gaps while novel sentences were being formulated, or that he is speaking pre-stored chunks of text. When at home, Peter mixes with a large extended family of speaking young people and their friends, and it is not hard to envisage the difficulties that he encounters using his communication equipment in fast-moving conversations.

Thomas *et al.* (1989) highlight the role of poor conversational skills and ability to 'mesh' (speaking without butting in or talking over) in their sample of young people with physical disability. These subjects had speech. In response to Peter's request, his speech and language therapist is investigating new software with him (*e.g.* Vocab Plus, developed by Liberator), to see if he will find it quicker to access a differently organized word-prediction-based communication programme.

Cockerill and Fuller (Chapter 4) have described the impact of a poor state of health, and an inadequate nutritional status, on the ability to use communication equipment effectively. Peter is underweight and frequently appears tired. It has been recommended, on the basis of videofluoroscopy evidence, that he have a gastrostomy but he has resisted this with the result that he continues to have periodic chest infections and has difficulty maintaining adequate fluid intake. His very caring parents, though concerned, support his right to make this decision.

Discussion

These case histories demonstrate that the process of assessment and monitoring must continue into adulthood to provide communication aids that meet the user's changing needs. Otherwise there is a risk that AAC equipment will become redundant or abandoned by the user. In addition to the influence of physical maturation, growth or, in some cases, degeneration, it is necessary to be aware of the young person's changing emotional responses to communication equipment in the adolescent years. There is a need for regular monitoring of usage, the availability of counselling, a constructive relationship between the adolescent and the staff who work with her/him, and an awareness of adolescent concerns and preoccupations. Communication equipment must be maintained, upgraded and reprogrammed. There should be tolerance for periods of apparent rejection of technology.

Speed may not be achievable. Communication may remain physically and/or cognitively demanding, with the result that the aid may be used only at certain times in the day. This means there is always a place for low-tech equipment. However, independently accessed, readily available, wheelchair-mounted voice output equipment can give the potential for even the non-literate user, to 'speak' to a wider range of communication partners. With it, communication becomes possible within groups, with young children, with the non-literate and with those who do not have the hand or eye control to access word boards and books. The user can call from room to room, speak on the telephone, and independently convey information.

Disabled adolescents with speech and language problems have been shown to be at increased risk of developing mental health problems. It is to be hoped that the provision of appropriate AAC systems and support will mitigate against this, by empowering the users, improving self-esteem, and enabling these young people to deal more effectively with their, often very complex, lives.

REFERENCES

Bodine, C., Beukerman, D.R. (1991) 'Prediction of future speech performance among potential users of AAC systems: a survey.' *Augmentative and Alternative Communication*, **7**, 100–111.

Castree, B.J., Walker, J.H. (1981) 'The young adult with spina bifida.' *British Medical Journal*, **283**, 1040–1042.

Coleman, J.C., Hendry, L. (1991) *The Nature of Adolescence*. London: Routledge.

—— Hertzberg, J., Morris, M. (1977) 'Identity in adolescence: present and future self concepts.' *Journal of Youth and Adolescence*, **6**, 181–185.

Davies, E., Furhham, A. (1986) 'Body satisfaction in adolescent girls.' *British Journal of Medical Psychology*, **59**, 279–287.

Harter, S. (1983) 'Developmental perspectives on the self system.' *In:* Hetherington, M. (Ed.) *Handbook of Child Psychology: Socialization, Personality and Social Development*. New York: Wiley, pp. 275–386.

Ireys, H.T., Werthamer-Larsson, L.A., Kolodner, K.B., Shapiro Gross, S. (1994) 'Mental health of young adults with chronic illness: the mediating effect of perceived impact.' *Journal of Paediatric Psychology*, **19**, 205–222.

Jessop, D., Stein, R. (1985) 'Uncertainty and its relation to the correlates of chronic illness in children.' *Social Science and Medicine*, **20**, 993–999.

Jolleff, N., McConachie H., Winyard S., Wisbeach, A., Clayton, C. (1992) 'Communication aids for children—procedures and problems.' *Developmental Medicine and Child Neurology*, **34**, 719–730.

Ko, M.L.B., McConachie, H., Jolleff, N. (1998) 'Outcome of recommendations for augmentative communication in children.' *Child: Care, Health and Development*, **24**, 195–205.

Mauldon, J. (1992) 'Children's risks of experiencing divorce and remarriage – do disabled children destabilize marriages?' *Population Studies – A Journal of Demography*, **46**, 349–362.

Pless, B., Stein, R.E.K. (1994) 'Intervention research: lessons form research on children with chronic disorders.' *In:* Haggerty, R.J., Sherrod, L.R., Garmezy, N., Rutter, M. (Eds.) *Stress, Risk and Resilience in Children and Adolescents*. Cambridge: Cambridge University Press, 317–353.

Rosenberg, M. (1979) *Conceiving the Self*. New York: Basic Books.

Seiffge-Krenke, I. (2000) 'Causal links between stressful events, coping style, and adolescent symptomatology.' *Journal of Adolescence*, **23**, 675–691.

Stein, R.E.K., Gortmaker, S.L., Perrin, J., Perrin, E.K., Pless, I.B., Walker, D.K. (1987) 'Severity of illness: concepts and measurements.' *Lancet*, **2**, 1506–1509.

Tatar, M. (1998) 'Significant individuals in adolescence: adolescent and adult perspectives.' *Journal of Adolescence*, **21**, 691–702.

Thomas, A.P., Bax, M.C.O., Smyth, D.P.L. (1989) *The Health and Social Needs of Young Adults with Physical Disabilities. Clinics in Developmental Medicine No. 106*. London: Mac Keith Press.

Walczak, Y., Burns, S. (1984) *Divorce: The Child's Point of View*. London: Harper & Row.

Wallerstein, J.S., Kelly, J.B. (1980) *Surviving the Breakup: How Children and Parents Cope with Divorce*. New York: Basic Books.

West, J, (1999) '(Not) talking about sex: youth, identity and sexuality.' *Sociological Review*, **47**, 525–547.

136

8
SUPPORTING AUGMENTATIVE AND ALTERNATIVE COMMUNICATION

Susan Balandin and Tessa Barnes-Hughes

Organization of AAC services: models of service delivery

When discussing models of augmentative and alternative communication (AAC) service delivery, it is tempting to focus on 'good practice' and models of service delivery that are likely to best meet the needs of children who use AAC and their families. Sadly, AAC service delivery is influenced by more than this. Although there is general agreement that AAC services are best offered using a team approach (Beukelman and Mirenda 1998, Lee Maher and Associates and Centre for Developmental Disability Studies 1998, Simpson *et al.* 1998), the funding of services and the geographic area in which they are delivered frequently affect the model of service delivery. In addition, there are a variety of team approaches that also impact on the model of service delivery employed. Thus, it is possible to define models of service delivery by the type of team approach, be it integrated or collaborative (Pugach and Johnson 1995, Giangreco 1996), interdisciplinary (Yorkston and Karlan 1986, Beukelman and Mirenda 1998) or transdisciplinary (Locke and Mirenda 1992).

The examples in this chapter are taken from Australian educational systems; readers from other countries will be able to apply the principles to the situation in their own settings. In metropolitan areas, AAC services may be offered by a specialist therapy team using one of the above approaches. The team may specialize in community health (generalist paediatric and adult clinical caseload), developmental disability, or AAC and assistive technology. Specialist developmental disability teams usually offer 'low-tech' AAC interventions and will refer individuals requiring 'high-tech' solutions to a specialist AAC team (Sigafoos and Iacono 1993). Traditionally, a developmental disability therapy team involves a speech pathologist, occupational therapist and physiotherapist as the core team, with access to the services of a paediatrician, psychologist, social worker and teacher for assessment and support of the child and family if required. Specialist AAC teams usually comprise a speech pathologist, occupational therapist and rehabilitation engineer. There is also general agreement that all models of service delivery should include the person who uses AAC and the parents or carers if that person is under 18 years old or requires additional support. In addition, the team should seek input from others who provide a service or have contact with the person who uses AAC, including teachers and peers and others who have specialist skills. This is particularly important for children with specific individual impairments (Giangreco 1996, Beukelman and Mirenda 1998, Lee Maher and Associates and Centre for Developmental Disability Studies 1998).

Although many services are attempting to use a collaborative or integrative approach to service delivery (Pugach and Johnson 1995, Giangreco 1996), therapists who have traditionally been responsible for making discipline-specific decisions on service delivery (Nesbit 1993) may experience difficulty in providing a service using a collaborative approach. In some rural areas there may be a lack of availability of therapists as a result of unfilled vacancies (Lee Maher and Associates and Centre for Developmental Disability Studies 1998), and so families may approach individual therapists working in the private sector or may have to rely on infrequent consultation with teams visiting the rural area from a metropolitan centre. Therapists working on nonspecialist teams or in private practice may not have expertise in AAC interventions or may have limited access to AAC information and resources (Balandin and Iacono 1998a). There are currently few reports on AAC services delivered using telecommunication equipment (Brodin 1996), but models of service using video-telephony hold great potential for service delivery and intervention (Lindstrom and Moniz Pereira 1995, Brodin 1996).

In Australia, most AAC services to children are funded by state government departments or non-governmental organizations (NGOs), with relatively few individuals gaining service through the private sector (usually from speech pathologists in solo private practice, or from private clinics attached to universities). Children with a severe communication impairment (SCI) rarely receive AAC services from speech pathologists employed in hospital departments. A few hospitals may have a specially funded department that provides AAC services to children, but most hospital departments in Australia are poorly resourced for AAC (Russell and McAllister 1995, Balandin and Iacono 1998a). As a consequence, children tend to be referred to a specialist AAC service external to the hospital or are occasionally visited by the specialist service while still in hospital. Such specialist services are often part of an NGO that primarily services individuals with cerebral palsy or those with an intellectual disability.

In the current climate of economic cutbacks, many NGOs that employ a specialist AAC team now provide a free or minimal cost service only to individuals who are members of the organization, and it is common practice to charge a fee of non-members who choose to access the AAC service offered by the organization. In addition, some AAC manufacturers offer a service to individuals who use the company's products, as well as training sessions in the use of AAC. Thus, AAC service delivery in many instances can be defined as a 'two tier model' in which the regular service (*e.g.* community health team, developmental disability team, private practitioner) implements some AAC interventions but refers children who require high-tech assistive technology, or those who have additional problems that may require a specialist approach (*e.g.* seating difficulties, assessment for computer access), to a specialist AAC team.

Models of AAC service delivery can also be described as 'three tier' (The Spastic Centre of New South Wales 1998). This model is similar to other models of service delivery worldwide in having differing levels of day-to-day involvement and expertise: primary, secondary and tertiary.

PRIMARY
Primary service is comprised of seven components that include (i) assessment; (ii) prescription,

design and customizing of AAC equipment, including mounting and integration with other systems; (iii) consultation and collaboration with other service providers (*e.g.* the education department; (iv) providing education and information to the person using AAC, the family and others closely involved; (v) coordination, case management and referral to other specialist services; (vi) planning, including participation in individuals' educational planning; and (vii) therapeutic intervention, including individual therapy and group therapy.

SECONDARY

Secondary services are those in which another service or agency is involved as the primary service provider. Thus, consultation services where the AAC service is requested to see a client (possibly for a second opinion) and make recommendations about management, providing information, reports or training to another agency or requests for a service to become involved in the planning and coordination of services for a specific client are considered secondary level services.

TERTIARY

Tertiary service delivery provides information and training to the wider community including other service providers, schools, employers and organizations. There is a focus on skills transfer, professional development and both undergraduate and postgraduate teaching.

It is clear that this model encompasses different modes of service delivery, all of which may be relevant at different stages of an AAC intervention. It also allows for a model of service delivery that can be used in areas where resources are limited, or where the individual using AAC lives far from where the AAC services are located. Thus, a child living in a rural area may receive an initial assessment (primary service), the AAC team may visit the area annually to work with the local therapist (secondary service), and teachers and other professionals may have the opportunity to attend in-service training on AAC, as part of their professional development programme (tertiary service). An important part of any support offered to indivduals who use AAC and their families is the support of the AAC team, who ensure that the communication device is mounted properly and also assist with integrating systems so that they can be used with optimal efficiency.

Supporting AAC: integration of AAC with other systems

Many people who use AAC systems may also need to use other forms of assistive technology such as wheelchairs, environmental control units (ECUs) or computer access devices. Often these systems need to be used concurrently with a communication device. Therefore, it is important to ensure that they work together and that the use of the augmentative device does not prevent the use of the wheelchair or other assistive technology. Similarly, it is important that, for example, the wheelchair can accommodate other assistive devices that an individual may require (Church and Glennen 1992).

There are several issues that impact on integrating AAC with other systems. One of the most important is the mounting of the device so that the person using the system can have access to it whenever needed. Another important consideration is whether the AAC system and any other assistive technology systems should be integrated into a single device.

ACCESS

Warwick (1998) noted that it is important to ensure that communication can occur anywhere, anytime. This is as true for a person using AAC as for natural speakers. She further noted that people who use AAC must be able to transport their systems easily. In addition, Blackstien-Adler *et al.* (1990) emphasized that in order for communication systems to be effective they must be accessible to the system user. The individual's ability to use the device whether by pressing a key or pointing to or looking at a symbol is termed access. Clinicians agree that there is a positive relationship between effective therapeutic positioning and access (*i.e.* those who are seated properly in their chairs or at a table are likely to be able to access their devices more easily). Consequently, AAC systems must be mounted in a way that facilitates trunk, hand, head and eye control in order to optimize the user's access.

Finding how best to enable the individual to carry her/his AAC system around and have it easily accessible at all times is an ongoing challenge for AAC teams. Seating and mounting systems are invariably customized for the individual and may include designing a mounting system for a wheelchair, desk or bed, or making a special carry bag so that the device is readily accessible when needed.

MOUNTING—WHAT TO CONSIDER

In order to mount an AAC system on a wheelchair the clinician needs to consider a range of factors. Clinicians aim to mount a system so that it is accessible and safe. For a wheelchair mount, the device must also be within the confines of the wheelchair and not impede the operation of the chair. Questions the clinician may need to ask before mounting any system may include:

- How is the system to be powered, from the wheelchair battery or through rechargeable batteries? If the latter, does the device need to be removed for charging?
- How does the person using the device move in and out of her/his wheelchair? The mounting system may need to be removable or to swing away so that it does not impede transfers.
- In a powered chair, can the communication device stay on the mount while the user is driving or does the user need to swing it out of the way while driving then reposition it when s/he wishes to communicate?
- Will a mount prevent or lessen the independence of the user performing other activities such as using their wheelchair tray or using a computer keyboard? Again does it need to swing away during these activities?

Commercial systems are available to mount AAC systems to wheelchairs. These mounts usually consist of a series of adjustable tubes, articulated joints and clamps that support a communication device at an optimal height, depth and angle. Many AAC device manufacturers make mounting plates to attach the devices to these commercial mounts. However, attaching a standard mounting is often not straightforward as wheelchairs vary considerably (Brown 1995). Sometimes the mount will need to be customized to meet the user's needs. Usually a person who uses AAC will consult a specialist team to gain advice and assistance with device mounting.

TRANSPORT

If the person who uses AAC is to travel in a bus, car or taxi it is important that the AAC device and mounting system are not safety hazards and at risk of becoming a projectile in the event of an accident. It is recommended that mounting systems and communication devices be removed from wheelchairs and well secured during transportation (Standards Australia 1994).

INTEGRATING VOICE OUTPUT AAC SYSTEMS WITH OTHER ELECTRONIC SYSTEMS

Assistive technology options for people with disabilities are increasing as more technology is developed. A person who uses an AAC system may wish to operate it alongside an ECU, call system or computer. This may necessitate the use of an integrated system. Guerette *et al.* (1994) described integrated systems as those where a single input device is used to access more than one assistive device. For example, a wheelchair joystick control could be used to drive the chair and operate a computer. This is possible using a wheelchair control box with different modes that allow different functions. The user may use one mode to drive the chair, then switch to a different mode that activates an infra-red transmitter; a receiver in the computer would then translate the joystick movements into cursor movements on the screen.

An integrated system may be considered for several reasons, for instance when the client has only one way to access both systems, or if s/he prefers an integrated system because it looks better or is less tiring to use (Guerette *et al.* 1994). An integrated system is likely to be easier to mount on a chair and be more portable than separate systems. For example, a student with a disability may need to take an AAC system and a device to record written work between classrooms at school. Independent access may be made significantly easier if both needs are met by a single system. Several AAC devices allow access to environmental control systems. They use a programmable infra-red transmitter that can learn the infra-red codes for different remote-control appliances such as a CD player or TV. Users are then able to have more independence, operating their own music, TV, doors and lights without assistance from a carer. Similarly, a range of voice output communication devices can be used as computer keyboard alternatives.

LAPTOP COMPUTERS AS INTEGRATED SYSTEMS

The proliferation of portable computers is expanding the possibilities for integration of several assistive technology systems in one device. It is possible to use a laptop with specialist software to run regular software alongside an AAC system and at the same time control an ECU. Using a regular laptop computer as an AAC system as opposed to a dedicated AAC device presents a set of challenges. Battery life on a laptop is too short to support an AAC system that needs to hold enough charge to be of use throughout the day. Those who use wheelchairs can circumvent a lack of sufficient battery charge by running the laptop from the wheelchair battery. The difficulty many people who use AAC systems face is how to open the lid and position the screen of the laptop independently. However, there are specialist portable computers on the market with built-in touch screens and no lid, that remove this problem.

Development of new AAC technology: funding and research

Sadly, it would seem that in most countries a coordinated, needs-based programme of research and development into new AAC devices does not exist. At present, product development is largely market driven, with most larger manufacturers spending a great deal of time and money on research and development that ensures that new products have a financially viable market. Consequently, most new AAC devices are developed and manufactured in the USA or UK where there is the population to purchase a profitable number of devices. Additionally, in the USA there is some legislation to support the use and therefore purchase of AAC devices. In contrast, in countries with a low population (*e.g.* Australia) the potential market is small and there may be no national funding agreement to supply devices for people with communication disabilities.

The lack of voice output devices that have different accents is very frustrating for those who use AAC and who see themselves as separate from the USA or UK. Although people may complain that they do not like the accent used on their communication device, there is little chance that manufacturers will produce devices that are tailored to individuals' cultural needs unless there is likely to be a large and profitable market for the product. In the case for example of Australia, it is unlikely that a device capable of producing an Australian accent will be developed as the population is too small. Similarly, regional variations of UK or North American English are not likely to be built in to communication devices.

In order to keep costs down, many manufacturers use mainstream components in their devices. If mainstream technology is not available then they may use technology developed for other markets. For example, the eye-movement recognition equipment that can guide a mouse cursor around a screen was originally developed for fighter pilots. Technology continues to be a rapidly growing area, yet the market for augmented communication devices and assistive technology remains relatively small. Consequently, many manufacturers are embracing 'universal design'. This is a concept where a product designed for a niche market such as the disability market has applications to the wider population. Products that have broad application will have high sales and the price is likely to be lower. Often, the most expensive components are those that have to be developed specifically for an individual product (*e.g.* custom-made plastic moulds). If a small firm invests in expensive components it may be difficult to change the design of a device. Rather than small firms attempting to address a niche market based on the needs of a few individuals known to them, it would seem imperative for research to inform the development of devices so that large manufacturers could develop devices that addressed a variety of needs.

Research grants to design and develop products rarely result in a finished product unless a commercial company becomes involved. Indeed, many products that benefit those who use AAC may not be available for use once the research project is completed. This raises ethical problems for researchers, and is also frustrating for those using AAC who are not able to keep a device that they may have used successfully in a research project (Alm 1994). A research team trialling a prototype device or system cannot supply the ongoing support and maintenance that is expected to be provided by a reputable manufacturer. Therefore it is considered unethical to provide a device that has no guarantee of working over a period of time and that cannot be repaired if it breaks down. Closer links between researchers and manufacturers remain problematic. Manufacturers are driven by market forces and are unlikely to want to participate in projects that do not promote their own device. In addition, if manufacturers fund their own research, it is difficult to argue that this work is not biased.

FUNDING

Funding for devices is a problem for many people in many countries. Indeed there are many individuals who could benefit from electronic communication devices, or who need customized chairs or equipment but are unable to purchase what they require. Just as there is limited funding for research and development, there is also limited funding for purchasing devices. Within any one country, the funding provision for devices may vary from region to region or state to state. Some countries will provide devices for children as long as they are in school (*e.g.* Canada), whereas in others there may be no funding at all. Frequently parents or carers must fund the purchase of devices or must approach charities. Many charities focus specifically on the needs of children and are prepared to fund communication devices and assistive technology for young and school-aged children but may not be prepared to provide technology for young or older adults.

Funding may be available through the public health or social service system. However, this funding may cover all equipment and consequently there may not be enough to purchase expensive communication devices. Similarly, those who allocate funding may choose to fund many small pieces of equipment for many people (*e.g.* 200 walking sticks) rather than a few pieces of expensive equipment. If the health service is responsible for funding equipment, much of the funding may be used for funding vital medical equipment (*e.g.* oxygen) leaving little for equipment that may not be deemed life saving or even necessary. It is almost incredible that augmented communication devices may be seen not as a priority but rather a luxury, but there are many places where this is still the case. The argument that low-tech devices (*e.g.* communication boards and books) are cheaper is specious. The cost of developing, mounting and maintaining such boards can be high as it involves not only materials but also a specialist's time. Such devices must be updated regularly and well maintained if they are to be useful, and over time this can be as costly as purchasing an electronic communication device.

Communication is recognized as a basic human right, therefore it is a matter of great concern that there are many people who do not have the technology, services or devices that they require in order for them to participate in communication and to obtain their best quality of life. Nevertheless, provision of a device and correct mounting alone will not ensure successful communication. Unless all those involved with a person who uses AAC receive adequate support and training in communication issues, that person may not develop optimal use of the device or of her/his communication skills.

Training and supporting families, teachers, carers, employers and the wider community

Any model of AAC service delivery must ensure that those who plan the service and those who deliver it provide support and training not only to the person who uses the AAC system, but also to other people who are closely involved (*e.g.* parents, teachers, peers). The focus of AAC interventions is to promote communication in natural contexts (Musselwhite and St.Louis 1988, Reichle *et al.* 1991, Marvin 1994, Balandin and Iacono 1998b, Beukelman and Mirenda 1998). Thus not only the close circle of family and friends but also members of the general community (*e.g.* employers and work colleagues, the proprietor of the local cafe, or staff in the supermarket) may also require some support and training in communicating with someone who uses AAC. Indeed, there is consensus in the literature that the skills required for a successful AAC interaction are different from those required for a communicative interaction between two natural speakers, and that these different skills may need to be taught (Calculator 1988, McNaughton and Light 1989).

Much has been written on training and support for communication partners and the wider community (*e.g.* Tatenhove 1987, Calculator 1988, Halle 1988, Musselwhite and St.Louis 1988, Goossens *et al.* 1992, Robinson and Owens 1995, Romski and Sevcik 1996, McConachie and Pennington 1997, McCall and Moodie 1998). Nevertheless, ensuring that communication partners have the skills to support those who use AAC and that the wider community is sympathetic to this group's needs remains an ongoing challenge for all those involved in the field of AAC. A number of surveys of speech pathologists' knowledge of AAC (Murphy *et al.* 1996, Russell and McAllister 1995, Balandin and Iacono 1998a, McCall and Moodie 1998, Simpson *et al.* 1998) have indicated that many speech pathologists lack expertise in AAC. When considering how best to provide support and training in AAC, it is imperative that the speech pathologists are well trained and competent in AAC so that they have both up-to-date knowledge on AAC and the confidence to impart skills to others (Balandin and Iacono 1998a, Simpson *et al.* 1998). Training in AAC for speech pathologists should be offered as part of undergraduate courses, with additional opportunities provided through postgraduate courses and ongoing professional development courses. Such training must include information and strategies for training and supporting the communication partners of individuals who use AAC systems to communciate.

If a collaborative or integrative model of service provision is used, parents, carers, family members and teachers will be involved in the whole AAC process. Thus, they will have opportunities not only to seek information but also to problem-solve and develop ideas as part of the AAC team. However, many families and support personnel are not involved in collaborative teams and may not be present at the time of AAC assessment or intervention. If those who communicate with and support the person who uses an AAC system are not trained in AAC, not only will social interactions suffer, but the whole AAC process may break down (Cumley and Beukelman 1992, Mirenda 1992).

The provision of support and training to families who live in remote rural areas, or to teachers in schools where therapy services are not provided in the school programme, may be problematic. Similarly, staff in tertiary education institutions and employers may have little if any experience with AAC. A recent study of access to technology by students with a physical disability (Balandin *et al.* 1999) revealed that those who support students (*e.g.* disability liaison officers, librarians) in universities and post-school vocational training centres have little knowledge of AAC. Because budgets are limited and knowledge of technology is often scant, the tertiary institution is more likely to provide an assistant to help the student rather than equipment to enable the student to work independently (Balandin *et al.* 1999). There may be limited equipment available, and the staff who are identified as supporting students with a disability, including those who use AAC, may have had little training in disability issues and no training in using, maintaining and helping with AAC devices or computer access technology. Balandin *et al.* (1999) recommended that any staff who have a responsibility for assisting students with a disability should be financially supported to attend workshops and training opportunities. Specialist services organize workshops and seminars, and some universities now offer AAC courses that are available in distance mode and are open to people who are not enrolled in degree courses. There are also a number of training courses and other resources available on the internet.

The internet is a useful resource both for people who use AAC and for those who support them. Many organizations [*e.g.* the International Society of Augmentative and Alternative Communication (ISAAC); the Australian Group on Severe Communication Impairment (AGOSCI); the United States Society for Augmentative and Alternative Communication (USSAAC); Communication Matters (ISAAC-UK)] have their own websites with links to other sites that have a focus on technology, disability and concomitant issues (*e.g.* literacy, health). In addition, there are a number of listservs, such as the Augmented Communication Online Users Group (ACOLUG) and those operated by AGOSCI and ISAAC), that provide an opportunity for online forums for discussion and problem-solving and that are used by people who use AAC, their parents and professionals.

The three-tier model of service delivery discussed above is a useful model for developing appropriate support services. We consider here a family with a 3-year-old female child who has cerebral palsy, who live in a rural area from which the nearest AAC specialist service is not easily accessible.

PRIMARY LEVEL SUPPORT

Initial support is offered at the primary level. The family come in to a specialist service in a metropolitan area for assessment, intervention and planning. The family are involved in the whole process as part of a collaborative team. Consequently, their goals and expectations are valued and considered. During the time that the family are at the service they have opportunities to discuss their needs with a number of professionals (*e.g.* physician, social worker, speech pathologist, occupational therapist) and there is also time for exploring specific concerns and attending other appointments (*e.g.* a dental check or a visit to the gait laboratory). The child is given an AAC system, in this instance a communication board and a simple single-message voice output device, and the family are taught how to use and maintain it and also what to do if it breaks down.

SECONDARY LEVEL SUPPORT

When the family return to the country, the specialist service team contact the local disability service providers (with the parent's permission) to discuss the child's intervention plan and management. The team provides recommendations about ongoing intervention and support, and provides relevant information to those who will be supporting the family in their home town. The specialist service forwards information and reports to the relevant professionals but still maintains responsibility for the overall management of the services. Staff from the service may also contact others who provide support (*e.g.* the local preschool teachers). When secondary level support services are being provided there may still be some ongoing primary support services (*e.g.* telephone consultations between staff from the specialist service and the family).

TERTIARY LEVEL SUPPORT

As noted above, tertiary service delivery provides information and support to the wider community. In the case of our rural family, the specialist service team decides to offer a short information session for rural general practitioners on communicating with patients who use AAC and also liaises with the Education Department to run a half-day workshop on implementing AAC in the classroom. The workshop is attended by preschool, infant and primary teachers and aides working in the education department in that region. These tertiary services are offered when the specialist service team goes on an annual visit to the area and offers primary support to the family.

Thus, it is clear that when support services function optimally, different levels of service may be offered concurrently. The local speech pathologist or a teacher may support the child in using her communication system in the community. Trips to the local shops, visits to the pool, as well as using the system in preschool provide opportunities for developing functional communication. The staff from the specialist service may provide ongoing support by sending symbols to support new vocabulary for the communication board if this is not available in the home town.

Johnson and Bloomberg (1990) noted that a shortage of qualified speech pathologists, a shortage of speech pathologists with appropriate expertise in AAC and a lack of direct service providers with knowledge of communicating with individuals with a severe communication impairment, all mitigated against those who require AAC receiving an appropriate service. They developed the Severe Communication Impairment Outreach Project (SCIOP) in Victoria, Australia (Johnson and Bloomberg 1990, 1991). SCIOP has provided training and support to thousands of people in Victoria and in other states of Australia. This may serve as a useful model in areas where AAC services are being established. SCIOP offers five types of consultancy: (i) face-to-face individual consultancy; (ii) assessment; (iii) group consultancy; (iv) phone and video consultancy; (v) consultancy with staff and carers.

Video consultancy is a cost-effective way of consulting with families who are living in remote areas and who cannot access services. A video is made of the individual with SCI and is sent to the SCIOP consultants with written information. Questions and concerns are included in the written information. The SCIOP consultants view the video, talk with the family or carers by telephone and then write a report listing recommendations and ideas. Subsequently, there may be additional telephone follow-ups.

SCIOP provides a range of training options that cover a variety of topics that relate to children or adults who cannot speak or are difficult to understand. Topics include alternatives to speech, sign and gesture, communication and challenging behaviour, communication and choice making and literacy. All training is competency based and involves pre-service consultation to ensure that the training is tailored to the needs of the trainees. This consultation involves visits to the site and observations of the individuals with SCI and discussions with the staff. Follow-up consultations occur approximately six weeks after the training. There are usually three follow-up consultancies, during which issues arising for individuals and general concerns are followed up. Training programmes such as this are a cost-efficient way of training a number of people and also ensuring that the training goals are met and put into practice.

Evaluation of the SCIOP model has indicated that not only have thousands of caregivers and teachers been trained using this model, but that those who have attended have been enthusiastic about this model of support and training (Johnson and Bloomberg 1990, 1991). It is resource-efficient and cost-effective, as the facilities contracting the service pay a fee but up to 65 people can attend the workshops.

AAC camps (Bruno 1996, Bruno and Dribbon 1998) also provide support and training to individuals who use AAC systems and their families. Such camps have additional benefits as they provide recreation and opportunity to increase social networks. As at all camps, there are opportunities for attendees to make new friends and experience new activities. Families have the chance to learn new skills and share experiences in a recreational setting.

Although there is a general agreement that there is still a shortage of speech pathologists with expertise in AAC (Balandin and Iacono 1998a), there are now a variety of means for people who use AAC systems and those who support them to gain training and expertise. Nevertheless, services to those with a severe communication impairment suffer from a lack of trained speech pathologists and funding to purchase necessary equipment and resources.

Schools may receive a lump sum of money to support the child with a disability. Usually the bulk of this money pays for the individual support assistant and there is little left to purchase special equipment and resources for use in the school. School therapists may often cover several schools and can spend little time with individuals or with the teachers and aides.

However, all is not totally bleak. Many countries now offer similar programmes to those described above. The wider community is becoming more aware of AAC and the importance of every member of the community having a functional communication system. Since the early 1970s, normalization and community integration (Nirje 1972, Wolfensberger 1972) has meant that people with a disability, including people who use AAC, are increasingly part of the general community. They are being educated in mainstream schools, are living and working in the community, and appear on television and in film. This, coupled with ever increasingly sophisticated communication technology has encouraged the development of programmes, videos and teaching modules to promote and support communication with those who use AAC.

People who use AAC are in full-time open employment, attending mainstream schools and universities, raising families and participating in the same community activities as their naturally speaking peers. People with a disability, including those with no or limited functional speech, are becoming increasingly vocal about their right to be valued by the community and to be in the community without having to strive to attain 'normality'.

147

AAC and the social model of disability

The social model of disability stresses that it is society that disables individuals deemed to have a disability by excluding them and restricting their full participation in the life of the community (Oliver 1996). Some therapeutic programmes (*e.g.* those that emphasize walking for those with a motor impairment, conductive education programmes) are heavily criticized for the assumption that people with a disability must strive to conform to society's view of normality (Oliver 1996). Prolonged speech therapy, focused on articulation skills, with no functional speech outcome rather than the provision of a suitable augmented communication system could be construed as oppression by service providers or those in a more powerful position than the individual with a severe combination impairment.

Despite the increased integration of people with a disability within the community, there is still a great deal of criticism from individuals who themselves have a disability that they must continue to battle with environments and community attitudes that are inherently 'disabling' (Oliver 1996). Disabling environments are composed of barriers to independence (Swain *et al.* 1996) and result in what Oliver (1996) terms 'social poverty'. Social poverty can be seen as exclusion from social activities and the same income-earning opportunities that are available to individuals in the community who are not deemed to have a disability. Oliver (1996) suggested that the education system has failed children with a disability as it has not taught or supported them to demand or accept the rights and responsibilities of being part of the wider community. In addition, those who provide services or conduct research in the field of disability have been accused of being oppressive and opportunistic (Abberley 1992, Oliver 1992, Swain *et al.* 1998). To date there is a paucity of literature that focuses issues and experiences that are specific to people who use AAC (Balandin and Raghavendra 1999). Nevertheless, it is possible to consider issues relevant to augmented communicators within the perspective of the social model of disability. In doing so we acknowledge that as we do not have a disability we write from our knowledge of issues discussed in the literature and related to us by people who use AAC rather than from any personal experience.

Individuals who use AAC educated in special schools, and indeed those educated in mainstream schools, frequently do not have equal access to the educational facilities available to their nondisabled peers. Problems of access and transport play a major role in preventing children with a physical disability enjoying the same freedom of movement around the school environment or that of tertiary education facilities (Pitt and Balandin 1995, Balandin *et al.* 1999). Students who do not have a functional communication system, or who are unable to access their communication aids at all times (*i.e.* in class and in recess), who are unable to access school buildings and playgrounds, and who do not participate in the same classes as their able-bodied peers are clearly not integrated into the education system. Children who attend special units in mainstream schools may never be perceived as belonging in the classes they attend for integrated lessons (Schnorr 1990). This lack of integration creates barriers to friendship and the social bonding that occurs between the other children in the mainstream class. In other words, the school experience, be it in mainstream or special school, may serve only to reinforce difference. Lack of literacy skills also has an impact on equality and acceptance within the community. Many people who use AAC have poor literacy skills, not necessarily because they are unable to learn to read, but rather because they either were never taught or because their education was disrupted by therapy sessions and a curriculum that did not follow that of their nondisabled peers.

Difference is signalled by visible signs (*e.g.* wheelchairs, communication aids) that are interpreted in different ways by other members of the community. Able-bodied individuals' interpretation of the implications of the communication aid that they see gives rise to actions that result in complaints that people who use AAC are 'talked down to' or shouted at as though deaf (Huer and Lloyd 1990, Balandin and Morgan 1997). Although there is a growing demand that difference should be not only accepted but also celebrated, emanating from people with disabilities themselves (Oliver 1996), nevertheless difference still results in marginalization within schools and in the wider community. People with a disability still experience problems with presenting a positive image. People who use AAC cite many examples of this (Williams 1993, Creech 1994). In a recent lecture, Allan (1999) who uses AAC noted that the language of disability is a language of care, of toilets and need. Employees who use AAC have also noted they have to work harder, longer, and apply for more positions than their nondisabled peers in similar jobs, and may still be overlooked or may work in jobs that are not concomitant with their qualifications.

It can also be argued that as long as labels such as 'disabled' or 'impaired' are in use, people (including those using AAC) will continue to be marginalized (Swain *et al.* 1996). The changing of labels (disability, impairment, developmentally delayed, retarded) may only serve to create confusion and do little to remove the negative connotations of difference. Indeed, Oliver (1996) defined disability as a 'socially imposed restriction'. In other words if there is no means of accessing services, equipment and funding without a label, be it severe communication impairment, physical disability or developmental disability, people will continue to seek a label in order to access services and consequently will be treated differently because of the label. Finkelstein (1996) noted any label of disability tends to result in decreased power and reduced economic status. This is certainly true for those who use AAC. A recent study by Balandin and Iacono (1997) suggested that within Australia there were only six employees who use AAC in full-time open employment; numbers in other countries appear to be also proportionally small (LaPlante 1993).

The research community has also been accused of contributing to the oppression of people with a disability (Oliver 1992, Zarb 1992). Few people who use AAC have participated in research as part of the research team, yet many have been research subjects (Balandin and Raghavendra 1999). As yet there is no research agenda set by people who use AAC, although they have reported on the benefits and positive experiences that come from being part of the research team (McGregor and Alm 1992). Individuals with a disability have a right to be included in all aspects of research (Oliver 1992, 1996; Zarb 1992; Ramcharan and Grant 1994; French and Swain 1997). Until research is directed by individuals with a disability, not only research validity but also the ideal of social equality remain a myth (Oliver 1992).

In conclusion, it would seem that there is little focus on AAC within the literature that considers the social model of disability, yet the issues raised within that literature are as applicable to those who use AAC as to any other group (*e.g.* people with a physical disability, the deaf community). The medical profession, service providers, researchers, planners and those who develop policies within the field of AAC may need to develop an awareness of how their actions might be construed as contributing to marginalization of people who use AAC rather than inclusion. Acceptance of difference rather than effort to 'normalize' is a key issue within the social model of disability. Ensuring that people who use AAC have access to the technology and communication systems they require, that they do not have to cope with physical access problems and that their environments are adapted so that they can function optimally will help reduce the oppression of difference and allow them the same rights to inclusion as are available to the general community.

REFERENCES

Abberley, P. (1992) 'Counting us out: A discussion of the OPCS disability surveys.' *Disability, Handicap and Society*, **7**, 139–155.

Allan, M. (1999) 'The language of augmented and alternative communication.' *ISAAC Bulletin*, **56** (May), 1–7.

Alm, N. (1994) *Ethical Issues in AAC Research*. Kerkrade, Holland: International Society of Augmentative and Alternative Communication (ISAAC), Jonkoping University Press.

Balandin, S., Iacono, T. (1997) *Impact of a Socially Valid Vocabulary on Interactions Between Employees with Severe Communication Impairment and their Non-disabled Peers. (Research Report 1)*. Canberra: Australian Government Publishing Co.

—— —— (1998a) 'AAC and Australian speech pathologists: A report on a national survey.' *Augmentative and Alternative Communication*, 239–249.

—— —— (1998b) 'A few well chosen words.' *Augmentative and Alternative Communication*, 14, 147–161.

—— Morgan, J. (1997) 'Adults with cerebral palsy: What's happening?' *Journal of Intellectual and Developmental Disability*, **22**, 109–124.

—— Raghavendra, P. (1999) 'Challenging oppression: augmented communicators' involvement in AAC research.' *In:* Loncke, F., Clibbens, J., Loyd, L.L. (Eds.) *Augmentative and Alternative Communication: New Directions in Research and Practice*. London: Whurr, pp. 262–277.

—— Smith, R., Gonzalez, D., Mackaway, J., Taylor, E. (1999) *Access to Technology by Students with a Physical Disability in Tertiary Education Institutions (Research Report)*. Sydney: Centre for Developmental Disability Studies.

Beukelman, D.R., Mirenda, P. (1998) *Augmentative and Alternative Communication: Management of Severe Communication Disorders in Children and Adults. 2nd Edn.* Baltimore: Paul H. Brookes.

Blackstien-Adler, S., Ryan, S., Naumann, S., Parnes, P. (1990) 'Development of an integrated wheelchair tray system for augmentative communication.' *Assistive Technology*, **2**, 142–150

Brodin, J. (1996) 'Communication and social interaction for persons with mental retardation by use of videotelephones.' *Paper presented at the 7th Biennial Conference of the International Society of Augmentative and Alternative Communication, Vancouver, August 7–10.*

Brown, D. (1995) *Mounting Communication Devices to Wheelchairs. 2nd Australian Conference on Technology for People with Disabilities*. Adelaide: The Crippled Children's Association of South Australia.

Bruno, J. (1996) 'Outcomes in AAC: Measuring the effectiveness of a parent training program.' *Paper presented at the 7th Biennial Conference of the International Society for Augmentative and Alternative Communication, Vancouver, August 7–10.*

—— Dribbon, M. (1998) 'Outcomes in AAC: Evaluating the effectiveness of a parent training program.' *Augmentative and Alternative Communication*, **14**, 59–70.

Calculator, S.N. (1988) 'Promoting the acquisition and generalization of conversational skills by individuals with severe disabilities.' *Augmentative and Alternative Communication*, **4**, 94–103.

Church, G., Glennen, S. (1992) *The Handbook of Assistive Technology*. San Diego: Singular Publishing.

Creech, R. D. (1994) 'Practical problems of employment: A personal view.' *Paper presented at the Pittsburgh Employment Conference, Pittsburgh, PA, August 12–14.*

Cumley, G.D., Beukelman, D.R. (1992) 'Roles and responsibilities of facilitators in augmentative and alternative communication.' *Seminars in Speech and Language*, **13**, 112–119.

French, S., Swain, J. (1997) 'Changing disability research: Participating and emancipatory research with disabled people.' *Physiotherapy*, **83**, 26–32.

Giangreco, M.F. (1996) *Vermont Independent Services Team Approach*. Baltimore: Paul H. Brookes.

Goossens, C., Crain, S.S., Elder, P.S. (1992) *Engineering the Preschool Environment for Interactive, Symbolic Communication*. Birmingham, AL: Southeast Augmentative Communication Conference Publications.

Guerette, P., Caves, K., Nakai, R., Sumi, E. (1994) *Determining the Appropriateness of Integrated Control of Assistive Devices*. Los Amigos Research and Education Institute, Rancho Los Amigos Medical Centre Annual Report.

Halle, J. (1988) 'Adopting the natural environment as the context of training.' *In:* Calculator, S., Bedrosian, J. (Eds.) *Communication Assessment and Intervention for Adults with Mental Retardation*. San-Diego: College-Hill, pp. 155–185.

Huer, M.B., Lloyd, L.L. (1990) 'AAC users' perspectives on augmentative and alternative communication.' *Augmentative and Alternative Communication*, **6**, 242–249.

Johnson, H., Bloomberg, K. (1990) 'Case study: SCIOP: The severe communication outreach project (Victoria).' *In:* Butler, S.R. (Ed.) *The Exceptional Child*. London: Harcourt Brace Jovanich, pp. 304–310.

—— —— (1991) 'Severe Communication Outreach Project.' *Communication Matters*, Summer 1991, 15–19.

LaPlante, M.P. (1993) 'Estimating the size of the speech-impaired population, use of speech aids and employment patterns.' *Paper presented at the Pittsburgh Employment Conference, Pittsburgh, PA, August 20–22.*

Lee Maher and Associates and Centre for Developmental Disability Studies (1998) *Review of Therapy Services*. Sydney: Ageing and Disability Department.

Lindstrom, J., Moniz Pereira, L. (1995) 'Videotelephony.' *In:* Roe, P.R.W. (Ed.) *Telecommunications for All* Brussels: Commission of the European Communities, pp. 110–118.

Locke, P., Mirenda, P. (1992) 'Roles and responsibilities of special education teachers serving on teams delivering AAC services.' *Augmentative and Alternative Communication*, **8**, 200–214.

Marvin, C.A. (1994) 'Cartalk! Conversational topics of preschool children en route home from preschool.' *Language, Speech, and Hearing Services in Schools*, **25**, 146–155.

McCall, F., Moodie, E. (1998) 'Training staff to support AAC users in Scotland: Current status and needs.' *Augmentative and Alternative Communication*, **14**, 228–238.

McConachie, H., Pennington, L. (1997) 'In-service training for schools on augmentative and alternative communication.' *European Journal of Disorders of Communication*, **32**, 277–88.

McGregor, A., Alm, N. (1992) 'Thoughts of a nonspeaking member of an AAC research team.' *Augmentative and Alternative Communication*, **8**, 153. *(Abstract.)*

McNaughton, D., Light, J. (1989) 'Teaching facilitators to support the communication skills of an adult with severe cognitive disabilities: A case study.' *Augmentative and Alternative Communication*, **5**, 35–41.

Mirenda, P. (1992) 'School to postschool transition planning for augmentative and alternative communication users.' *Seminars in Speech and Language*, **13**, 130–142.

Murphy, J., Markova, I., Collins, S., Moodie, E. (1996) 'AAC systems: obstacles to effective use.' *European Journal of Disorders of Communication*, **31**, 31–44.

Musselwhite, C.R., St.Louis, K.W. (1988) *Communication Programming for Persons with Severe Handicaps: Vocal and Augmentative Strategies. 2nd. Edn.* Boston: College-Hill Press.

Nesbit, S.G. (1993) 'Direct occupational therapy in the school system: When should we terminate?' *American Journal of Occupational Therapy*, **47**, 845–847.

Nirje, B. (1972) 'The right to self determination.' *In:* Wolfensberger, W. (Ed.) *The Principle of Normalization in Human Services*. Toronto: National Institute on Mental Retardation, pp. 176–193.

Oliver, M. (1992) 'Changing the social relations of research production.' *Disability, Handicap and Society*, **7**, 101–114.

—— (1996) *Understanding Disability*. London: Macmillan.

Pitt, S., Balandin, S. (1995) *Integration: Benefits and Problems*. Adelaide: The Crippled Children's Association of South Australia.

Pugach, M.C., Johnson, L.J. (1995) *Collaborative Practitioners Collaborative Schools*. Denver: Love Publishing.

Ramcharan, P., Grant, G. (1994) 'Setting one agenda for empowering persons with a disadvantage in the research process.' *In:* Rioux, M., Bach, M. (Eds.) *Disability is Not Measles: New Research Paradigms in Disability*. Ontario: Roeher Institute, pp. 227–244.

Reichle, J., York, J., Sigafoos, J. (1991) *Implementing Augmentative and Alternative Communication: Strategies for Learners with Severe Disabilities*. Baltimore: Paul H. Brookes.

Robinson, L.A., Owens, J.R.E. (1995) 'Clinical notes: Functional augmentative communication and positive behavior change.' *Augmentative and Alternative Communication*, **11**, 207–211.

Romski, M.A., Sevcik, R.A. (1996) *Breaking the Speech Barrier: Language Development Through Augmented Means*. Baltimore: Paul H. Brookes.

151

Russell, A., McAllister, S. (1995) 'Use of AAC by individuals with acquired neurologic communication disabilities: Results of an Australian survey.' *Augmentative and Alternative Communication*, **11**, 138–146.

Schnorr, R. F. (1990) '"Peter? He comes and goes . . .": First graders' perspectives on a part-time mainstream student.' *Journal of the Association for Persons with Severe Handicaps*, **15**, 231–240.

Sigafoos, J., Iacono, T. (1993) 'Selecting augmentative communication devices for persons with severe disabilities: Some factors for educational teams to consider.' *Australia and New Zealand Journal of Developmental Disabilities*, **16**, 133–146.

Simpson, K.O., Beukelman, D.R., Bird, A. (1998) 'Survey of school speech and language service provision to students with severe communication impairments in Nebraska.' *Augmentative and Alternative Communication*, **14**, 212–221.

Standards Australia (1994) *Wheelchair Occupant Restraint Assemblies for Motor Vehicles*. Canberra: Australian Government Printing Services.

Swain, J., Finkelstein, V., French, S., Oliver, M. (Eds.) (1996) *Disabling Barriers – Enabling Environments*. London: SAGE.

—— Heyman, B., Gillman, M. (1998) 'Public research, private concerns: ethical issues in the use of open-ended interviews with people who have learning difficulties.' *Disability and Society*, **13**, 21–36.

Tatenhove, G.V. (1987) 'Training caregivers and facilitators to select vocabulary: Implementation strategies for improving the use of communication aids in schools.' *In:* Blackstone, S.W., Cassatt-James, E.L., Bruskin, D.M. (Eds.) *Augmentative Communication: Implementation Strategies*. Rockville, MD: American Speech–Language–Hearing Association, pp. 6.30–6.42.

The Spastic Centre of New South Wales (1998) *School Age Program Manual*. Sydney: The Spastic Centre of New South Wales.

Warwick, A. (1998) Communication Without Speech: *Augmentative and Alternative Communication Around the World*. Toronto: ISAAC Press.

Williams, M.B. (1993) 'My first job interview.' *Paper presented at the Pittsburgh Employment Conference, Pittsburgh, PA, August 20–22*.

Wolfensberger, W. (1972) 'Additional implications of the normalization principle to residential services.' *In:* Wolfensberger, W. (Ed.) *The Principle of Normalization in Human Services*. Toronto: National Institute on Mental Retardation, pp. 1–17.

Yorkston, K., Karlan, G. (1986) 'Assessment procedures.' *In:* Blackstone, S. (Ed.) *Augmentative Communication: An Introduction*. Rockville, MD: American Speech–Language–Hearing Association, pp. 163–196.

Zarb, G. (1992) 'On the road to Damascus: First steps towards changing the relations of disability research production.' *Disability, Handicap and Society*, **7**, 125–138.

9
EXPERIENCES OF CHILDREN AND FAMILIES WHO USE AUGMENTATIVE AND ALTERNATIVE COMMUNICATION

Compiled by Gillian Hazell, Lesley Carroll-Few and Helen Cockerill

Leon's story

By Leon's mother

Leon's speech and eating development were affected by athetoid cerebral palsy from when he was very young. This I found very frustrating and upsetting. I thought my son and I would never be able to have a mother and son conversation. At this stage I would guess what he wanted to say, and ask him questions that needed a yes or no answer. His understanding was normal and he could nod and shake his head for yes and no. He spent a lot of time crying from frustration.

When Leon was 18 months old he was referred to The Cheyne Centre in London, a centre that specializes in children with cerebral palsy. One of his problems was vomiting after feeds. Leon had a fundoplication that stopped him from regurgitating. The operation was a success and Leon was much happier as a result. Leon attended the Centre regularly and work on his communication began.

• *Picture cards.* At first Leon was encouraged to make eye contact and point to pictures of his choice with his eyes. This enabled Leon to communicate what he wanted, but I still wanted him to speak. I felt I was always asking him questions and guessing what he wanted to say. Although the pictures gave us only limited conversation, they did help us to communicate.

• *Blissymbols.* As Leon's ability with pictures developed he was introduced to the Blissymbol system. Leon communicated well with the symbols and they provided him with a much greater vocabulary. Leon continued to try hard to speak and I think he saw himself as a speaker. I was beginning to understand his unintelligible sounds and his gestures as well as using his Blissymbols with eye-pointing. "Drink" and "eat" were the only things the whole family could understand.

• *RealVoice.* The next stage was when Leon was introduced to an electronic communication aid called a RealVoice. This gave him a lot more independence. It was programmed with vocabulary for his specific needs and contained a lot of things Leon wanted to say. Leon knew how to add and remove sentences himself. I did not like the robotic voice.

• *Cameleon with EZ Keys.* This device provided Leon with greater independence. It enabled him to do all his schoolwork independently, including examinations. It also provided him with back-up to his speech.

• *Portable Lightwriter with keyguard.* As Leon's mother I feel this is a fantastic invention! The Lightwriter can be taken everywhere as a back-up to Leon's speech. The device can be preprogrammed with topics for conversation or can be used for ongoing conversation. The voice is still American-sounding and robotic. Communication aids have certainly come a long way but the voice still needs improving. An English accent might do the trick.

From what I have written it can be seen how many different communication systems and technological devices have been necessary to help Leon to develop as the efficient communicator he now is.

Leon's speech has improved immensely. We are now able to have a mother and son conversation. We talk about everything, including girls. In the past I wanted Leon to have speech therapy to exercise his speech muscles. I thought speech exercises would enable Leon to talk clearly. It was hard to believe the speech therapists when they said my son would need a back-up for his speech. They were right.

When Leon was very young I was not interested in other methods of communication because I wanted Leon to speak. I soon realized that Leon really did need a back-up system to enable him to communicate well. This helped him to make sure his needs were met and his thoughts and feelings were understood. The frustration caused to the disabled person and his family can be heartbreaking and causes great misery to all concerned.

I would like to thank the specialist speech and language therapists for giving Leon a good start in his early life with his speech and communication. I can honestly say that I am now proud of how well Leon is communicating today with his speech, backed up with technology.

Matthew's story: Communication for children with severe physical and visual impairment
By Sally Townend, Matthew's Occupational Therapist*

In the field of AAC the majority of approaches are based on vision (*e.g.* symbols), touch (*e.g.* objects of reference) or movement (*e.g.* signing). For many systems a combination of these is required. However, if an individual has severe visual and physical impairments these approaches are limited and auditory skills need to be utilized.

This case study explores the development and use of '*auditory scanning*' with Matthew, who has severe cerebral palsy and a cortical visual impairment, as an approach to give him a formal system of communication.

When Matthew was 5 years old, staff working with him felt that his understanding was greater than he was able to express, although he was classified as having profound and multiple learning disabilities. Matthew's physical impairments are such that he has minimal fine and

*ACE Centre – North, Oldham, England.

gross motor control, which precludes the use of any tactile or movement communication systems, *e.g.* objects of reference. He is also registered blind with his only visual response being to a bright light source, precluding the use of any visual communication systems, *e.g.* symbols.

Although Matthew uses a selection of communication strategies including facial expression, vocalization and his "yes" response (which is a combination of facial expression and vocalization), a more formal system of communication would need to make use of his intact sense of hearing and be accessed via switches.

Matthew's only method of independent control over his environment is via the use of switches. His most effective access method is a switch controlled by his head. For Matthew to use a voice output communication system in the future he would need to develop excellent switching skills. To develop these skills Matthew had the opportunity to use his switch with a range of motivating activities including a vibrating cushion, tape recorder and BIGmack (a single message voice output communication aid) to deliver instructions such as "blow a raspberry". The battery-operated devices were used with a timer unit, so for one switch press he gained a predetermined length of reward. Using his switch Matthew demonstrated good anticipation skills, using a BIGmack to join in stories with a repeated phrase.

While Matthew continued to develop his switching skills, a more formal system of low-tech communication was introduced as he demonstrated good understanding of spoken language and the desire to communicate. Those who worked with Matthew already used direct speech to give him choices between two options; he would indicate his choice with his "yes" response. This is known as 'partner-assisted auditory scanning'. However, this method followed no consistent pattern, so it was hard for Matthew to predict what was coming next and made him reliant on the communication partner offering the option he required.

A low-tech communication book was set up to try to overcome some of these difficulties, and provide Matthew with a more formal approach to his communication. The book was set up using a branching technique to contain categories, subcategories and then the individual vocabulary items. The structure of the book was based on the Chailey Heritage communication system.

There was discussion between all team members involved on the organization of vocabulary to ensure effective mapping to allow for vocabulary expansion, without having to totally reorganize. There was concern whether we were organizing it logically from an auditory perspective versus a visual one. Matthew accesses this book by using partner-assisted auditory scanning, where the communication partner reads out the categories, subcategories and individual vocabulary items, waiting at each stage for Matthew to indicate his choice using his "yes" response.

Matthew's switching skills and ability to follow a partner-assisted auditory scan were then combined, using a computer. Switch Clicker, a programme that allows the creation of on-screen grids containing words, was used. The words could be scanned with an auditory prompt, allowing each word to be spoken in turn. The switch method used initially was a simple two-switch scan that allowed the programme to move to the next option every time Matthew pressed his switch, and he would hear the choice spoken. Initially a grid consisting of four choices of motivating activities that Matthew could receive immediately was set up. If Matthew heard the option he wanted he vocalized to indicate his choice, and this was responded to immediately. Matthew demonstrated very quickly that he had the understanding to make clear choices, consistently choosing his two favourites "chocolate" and "blow a raspberry" from the grid. We initially set the scan to be a two-switch scan, so Matthew could be in control of the speed items were spoken until he had a clear understanding of what was expected of him.

Matthew progressed very quickly to using an automatic auditory scan, where the computer spoke the choices automatically and he pressed his switch when he heard his choice. Matthew had the opportunity to access a range of grids to communicate and assist with his educational work.

With a voice output communication system in mind, Switch Clicker grids that linked together were set up. This allowed the front grid to give a choice of categories, which, if selected, linked to a grid of choices within that category. Matthew was quickly able to navigate his way around this to answer questions.

Therefore the appropriate voice output communication aid was investigated. The features that were considered important were:

- the ability to enable the strategy of 'branching' to make use of categories, subcategories and individual vocabulary, already used within the Clicker programme and in his low-tech communication book;
- the ability to auditory scan;
- the ability for the auditory scanning prompts to be spoken through a separate speaker/earphone in a different voice and volume to the voice for the spoken message;
- portability to allow mounting onto his wheelchair.

The DynaVox 2 voice output communication aid was identified as the most appropriate for Matthew.

After having the DynaVox 2 for a relatively short period of time Matthew started to use it for functional communication, on one occasion introducing himself to a sister's friend whom he recognized as a new person in his house.

Through our work with Matthew it has become clear that we need to consider whether children with multiple disabilities are missing the opportunity to develop a communication system because the focus is often placed on the development of their physical and visual skills.

As 56 per cent of children with visual impairments have additional disabilities*, this area needs to be investigated further to determine how best to develop and organize vocabulary to optimize auditory scanning, and determine strategies to use in developing auditory scanning systems with individuals like Matthew.

Shaun's story

*By Lilo Seelos, Shaun's Speech and Language Therapist***

I first met Shaun when he was eight-and-a-half years old and placed in a school for children

---

*RNIB (1992) *Blind and Partially Sighted Children in Britain: the RNIB Survey.* London: HMSO.
**Radlett Lodge, Radlett, England.

with autism. I observed him in his classroom during a group 'drinks time'. He was sitting in front of an A4 board onto which had been stuck blurred photographs of biscuits and cups. Shaun was expected to hand over a picture in exchange for the represented item. At that time Shaun's responses were considered by his teachers to be random. Further observation of Shaun in the classroom, and discussion with his teacher and learning assistants indicated he was a 'difficult' child who presented many unacceptable behaviours. These included climbing furniture, trying to help himself to meet his own needs and wants, being generally uncooperative, stripping, running from the room and being reluctant to engage in positive or constructive interaction with other people. This resulted in Shaun missing out on learning opportunities, and caused general frustration to both staff and Shaun. My remit was to provide some one-on-one input to Shaun with the aims of encouraging an acceptance of adult involvement, and increasing participation in classroom learning tasks.

Once individual sessions were initiated it became clear that while Shaun had no demonstrable understanding of spoken language, he did have strong visual skills. He had no difficulty in recognizing and understanding Rebus or Picture Communication Symbols representing concrete everyday objects and activities. Shaun responded well to symbolic work schedules and became increasingly interactive as he was able to predict the format and content of the sessions.

Classroom staff were encouraged to support their (simplified) spoken language with symbols and other picture materials. Shaun's response to this strategy was very positive. He gradually became more cooperative and accepting of adults wanting to work with him, enabling him to engage in an increasing range of learning tasks.

Shaun also responded well to the introduction of the Picture Exchange Communication System (PECS). This initially required Shaun to initiate requests by selecting an appropriate symbol and placing it in an adult's hand. He then progressed to combining the symbols for "I want" and the desired item. Shaun quickly and spontaneously generalized this skill from therapy sessions into the classroom setting: on one occasion, when I was late for a session, he combined the symbols "I want" and "work with Lilo" from his timetable, and gave the message to his teacher.

Since those initial sessions Shaun has been developing into a more competent and confident communicator who displays increasing enjoyment in interaction. He visibly wants to learn once he understands what a task is about. Using symbols his teacher found that he was able to understand the concept of 'healthy' and 'unhealthy' foods and had no difficulties sorting pictures of different foods into the appropriate categories.

Shaun's behaviour has improved markedly since he has been able to communicate his wants and needs. He will now use the symbols to ask to go to the toilet rather than trying to run out of the room. He has stopped climbing furniture and appears calmer and happier. He accepts he cannot always have what he asks for, possibly because he knows his message has been understood and acknowledged. He is generally more cooperative and enjoys interactive learning. His mother reports similar progress at home and is excited at having found a way of communicating successfully with Shaun. It has also made it easier to take Shaun to different places in the community.

There are still moments when Shaun can display 'difficult' behaviour, possibly when he does not have a symbol available to support communication. An example of this occurred when Shaun had completed some work in the residential unit of the school where he stays as a weekly boarder. Aware that it was the end of the school day, Shaun had run from the workroom to the lounge and put his slippers on. His learning support assistant wanted Shaun to return to the school to collect his bag. She used minimal language when trying to explain this to Shaun but Shaun protested strongly, dropping to the floor and refusing to return to the school. Eventually a symbol for 'bag' was produced and Shaun immediately got up, ran back to his classroom, collected his bag and returned to the residential unit independently.

Using symbols to supplement spoken language has increased Shaun's understanding of the world around him, has made learning tasks more accessible and has given him greater independence. It has enabled him to make clear spontaneous requests without having to rely on adults to interpret his behaviour. It has also made him calmer, less frustrated and a less frustrating child to be with.

Shaun now also uses symbols when he comes to the weekly tuck shop session. Shaun is very particular about which colour sweets he likes. He used to jump on the table if he could not see the sweet he wanted. Now he is happy to wait his turn and competently uses symbols to buy his sweets. He is more accepting when the sweet he had in mind is not available, and is beginning to choose different food items (including raw carrot!) instead.

David's story
By David, with help from his mother

I'm David and I am fourteen. I was two years old when I came to live with my family and they had been told that I wouldn't ever learn anything because my brain was too damaged, but somehow they couldn't agree with this. One day, after I'd been with them some months, Mum asked me if I could see a window? It took me ages to get my head round but when I found it she said my eyes sparkled! Then she asked me to find the television and I did. Then, wherever we were, Mum or Dad would ask me if there was a clock? Or was there a window? And one day we showed the Consultant that I could do this, so he said I had to be educated! Wowee!!

After this I went to several different playgroups at the hospital, and when I was three I started at my first school. This was a small unit attached to our local hospital and it seemed I had a lot to learn—and people there seemed to think I could. The days of being a vegetable were gone!! It was here that I started using the Blissymbol language. They gave me two flash cards with Blissymbols—one said "yes" and the other said "no" and suddenly I could have a say about what happened!! I could make choices.

When I was about four I went for an assessment at the ACE Centre in Oxford with Mum and Dad and my teacher. When we got there, I was put in front of a computer and given a hand switch and told that if I pressed it, something would happen! And it did!! I made lots of things happen and then I was given a second switch to use with my head. Now I could really show that I understood and knew what I was doing.

After about three years I moved on to a bigger school. It was OK at first, but later on my technology seemed to cause a bit of a problem there. I was using a RealVoice and

Scanpac at this time and it had to be set up on my chair, plugged in and switched on for me. Somehow things didn't always seem to come together. Sometimes it was fixed on my chair, but not switched on; or the RealVoice was switched on but my switches weren't plugged it. It was very frustrating and I did resent being thought stupid. It's very difficult sometimes when you can't speak and you are working with someone who just doesn't pick up your signals, or who just doesn't seem to expect you to do anything anyway. When this happens, after a while you get bored and fed up. What's the point of bothering when they don't understand? It's hard enough anyway.

About this time we asked for an update of my educational statement, and the Educational Psychologist was great. We talked about sport and things on the news and he had me eye-pointing words and spelling and lots more. His report said lots of things about my understanding, including the fact that although I couldn't speak in sentences I understood very quickly whether or not someone understood me.

Finding the equipment is really important and it does take a lot of time. Sometimes things look good in a brochure, or even when you see someone else using them, but that doesn't mean they are right for everyone! I've tried seating and wheelchairs that in theory are right for me, but in practise don't help me at all. I think my 8+8 and Cameleon are two of the best things. My 8+8 is a small box fixed to my wheelchair. I've had it about four years now and with it I can drive, access my Cameleon to speak, use my word processor, and access my painting programme, games and printer. It has also got a buzzer on it and some infra-red switches. It's good. We are getting things together. The only slight problem is that at present it takes me eight seconds to get into speech mode from driving. So, when I drive up to people they must give me time to get into speech mode!

Switches are another problem. I've tried using one, two or three! I've tried accessing them with my hands, or head, and anything else! However good they are, if I can't apply enough pressure, or if they can't be sited in the right place for me to access, they have to go! Once, I tried a new head support. It was really good. It helped me to sit so well. My back was straight and my head was supported really well. The problem was, I was so well supported I couldn't access my switches properly to speak or drive! It caused problems getting in and out of my seating as well, but, more importantly, I need to tilt my head to access my switches and this head support just didn't allow me to do that. You could perhaps change your method of access, but I can't. And then, the best switches are no good unless you've got the right computer, and that's no good without the right software, and none of it is any good without the right teacher! And so it goes on! Life is never dull or routine.

I have to use head switches for my communication, driving, word processor and so on, but I can't operate my CD games on my desktop this way. So, when I play cricket, Mum or Dad tie the joystick onto my chair so I can wrap my arm around it, and then I can bowl. I've got a Grand Prix game too, and one day I told Mum "right side". At first she didn't understand what I meant, but I made her understand that I wanted to access the right-hand side of my keyboard. I knew that if I could get to the keyboard I could control the cars, alter the settings, and the camera positions, and lots more. I know what I want to do and which keys I want to press, but my fingers won't do it. Now my wheelchair is positioned side-on to the keyboard and I get to it with my right hand because that is my best side. It's good fun. You've just got to do as much as you can. Anyway you can!

I've got about eighty-eight pages on my Cameleon at present. A lot of them are useful and have preprogrammed sentences—the sort of things I use a lot—about food, things I want to do, places I need to go, and that sort of thing. I've got a 'social' page that's useful when I meet new people—the "What's your name? Where do you live? What do you like doing?" sort of things. It's much easier and quicker to have a whole page for some topics. My real interest is sport so I've got a whole page for Grand Prix racing, premier league football and general sport as well!! There's no way we could programme every sentence I might want to use, so I have pages of nouns, verbs, describing words, feelings, colours, alphabet and so on, so I can make up my own sentences which is useful. When I'm doing this I use a sort of 'shorthand'. I'll give you an example of what I mean. If I was to build the sentence, word by word, to say "Can we go to town on Saturday?" it would mean using my head switch sixty-two times. Yes, sixty-two times! That's hard work and takes a long time. Don't worry! I don't do it! If I say "town Saturday" it is much quicker and only takes nineteen switch movements. Guess which I say? Wouldn't you? And of course if I sneeze when I'm saying something that means a lot more work because I hit the switch at the wrong time and lose my place!

I like the Cameleon because I can get my point across to people and say what I want to say—not necessarily what people think I want to say. And I can argue if I don't agree. I do get mad when people don't give me time, and when they think they know what I was going to say. How can they?

I told you I can argue with people now I have my Cameleon. One day I had an argument with Mum, and I won! I asked her if we could go to the computer shop on Saturday and buy a new CD for my computer. We went down and I had to decide whether I wanted a football game or a cricket game. I chose FIFA football. It was OK but the sound wasn't really right. Something was incompatible. On the next Thursday I asked Mum if we could go and get a new game, but she said "no" because they were too expensive and I'd just had one. I said the football game was old, but she said it wasn't. I said it was broken, but she said it wasn't really, just that the sound wasn't quite right. I said "please, please, please" but she said "no". I really didn't think I was going to win but I suddenly remembered something else I had stored in my Cameleon. We had done a shopping project in our communication group at school. It was ages ago but I knew it was there. I said "Please will you take the money out of my purse?" She was so surprised that she said "yes!" So I got Ian Botham's International Cricket game too! It's really great!!

Everyone is different and people like me are all different too. Some, like me, have problems with our output but we do not have problems with input. We hear, and understand. Sometimes more than we should! Some people think we are thick and deaf just because we are stuck in a wheelchair and can't speak like them. So often they don't see us, just our problems, our high-tech wheelchairs, our speech computers, and all the rest of it, and they don't un-derstand. I can accept that people don't know how my equipment works. It is complicated. But I do object, very much, when they suggest I am stupid when it is in fact them, just because they don't understand. And then sometimes they expect us to perform, just like a performing seal. We are not 'actors', playing a part. We are us. Not from choice, but because that's the way it is. And another thing—people must give us TIME. It takes TIME to get into speech mode. TIME to scan through our set-ups. TIME to get the words we want. TIME to compose our sentences. TIME to say it. Give us that TIME, and remember too how tiring it is. Remember, sixty-two head switch presses for seven words. Lastly, please don't 'talk down' to us. We are not simple. We understand. Often more than people think. And physically don't talk down to us either. You all talk face to face, with eye contact and facial expression. Why must we be different? If we're in a wheelchair sit down, or at least come to our level. We don't like talking to giants!

10
COMMUNICATION RESOURCES

Gillian Hazell and Helen Cockerill

Most of us assist our communication in some way by gesture, arm-waving, facial expression or other body language. Where speech is delayed, difficult to understand or absent, these supplementary means of communication become even more important. People with disordered speech may require more formal systems with which to augment their verbal or vocal communication.

This chapter focuses on the options available to those with communication impairments. 'Unaided communication' refers to communication methods that require no external device for production (*e.g.* manual signs). 'Aided communication' refers to those "which require some type of external assistance such as a device for production" (*e.g.* pictures and photographs, graphic symbols) (Beukelman and Mirenda 1992). This includes the use of sign languages and sign vocabularies, the use of graphic symbol sets and systems, and the use of voice output communication aids (VOCAs).

The need for individual augmentative and alternative communication (AAC) systems needs to be balanced against the needs of the people communicating with the individual, but the needs of the communication partners should not be the overriding concern. There are some basic considerations when selecting an AAC system for an individual user:
• *appropriateness* for the user's current linguistic, cognitive and manual skills
• *flexibility* to provide for development and growth
• *acceptability* of the AAC system to the community (family, school, etc.)
• *recognition of the user's need for an AAC system* by the user and the community.

When considering the introduction of an AAC system to an individual, it is essential that all aspects of the individual's needs are considered, such as:
• physical abilities—seating and access issues
• cognitive abilities
• sensory skills—hearing, vision, perceptual skills
• the environment and expectations within the environment
• access to the curriculum, later employment and recreation.

Manual systems

Most basic emotional and social body language is instinctive. Gesture is more ritualized and varies culturally. Almost everybody uses gesture to a greater or lesser extent when talking. Sign languages have developed within deaf communities. These are complete languages with little relation to the spoken language of the hearing community. Sign systems are artificially created to support the learning of spoken language. They often include formal compilation of gestures and specifically created signs to develop vocabulary. Sign sets are a selection of vocabulary (which may include individual signs from a sign language) that are used to sign the keywords of a spoken message.

Points to consider when selecting a manual system include:

- Are the signs transparent, *i.e.* easy to understand, so that, for instance, the sign for 'drink' looks like what it represents?
- Are the signs easy to make, *i.e.* are the hand shapes simple or complex?
- Are one or two hands necessary?
- Are signs symmetrical (both hands making the same shape and movements) or asymmetrical (one hand making one movement in one position and the other making a different movement in a different position)? Can the user move her/his hands in two different movements and positions?
- Which system will be used to meet the user's communication needs in the foreseeable future?
- Can additional vocabulary be obtained from a similar sign language, system or set if necessary?

SIGN LANGUAGES, SYSTEMS AND VOCABULARY SETS

The sign language used in the deaf community of the UK is British Sign Language (BSL). In the USA American Sign Language (ASL) is used. Neither of these correspond to spoken English, but each has its own grammar. Facial expression, body positions and postures are implicit in the use of sign languages and form part of the meaning of the utterances being signed. Finger spelling is a useful addition to BSL and ASL. There are dialectal variants of the language throughout the country, so in the UK some signs that are used in Cornwall, for example, will not be understood in Newcastle. Many countries have their own sign languages that have developed within the deaf community.

BSL forms the basis for a number of sign vocabularies, such as the Makaton Vocabulary and Signalong. These vocabularies take their signs from BSL and use them in English word order. Signs used in this way are often referred to as 'sign supported English'. Signed English also takes its signs from BSL, but has specially created signs for grammatical words and markers that do not exist in BSL vocabularies or BSL itself. For example, it is possible to sign the sentence "I went to see my sister's new puppies yesterday" so that it is signed as it is written or spoken, whereas in sign supported English one would sign "I go [perhaps 'went' might be used] see sister new baby dog [possibly 'dogs'] yesterday". The complexity of the signed utterance would depend on the user's knowledge of signing.

Sign vocabularies differ in their size, the vocabulary they represent and their organization. The Makaton Vocabulary was originally developed in the early 1970s for use with deaf adults with severe learning difficulties in a hospital environment in the UK. The vocabulary has increased greatly and now there are approximately 1600 signs and symbols in total (450 in the Core Vocabulary, 600 in the National Vocabulary and about 500–600 in the first section of the Resource Vocabulary). The Makaton Vocabulary is widely used with children and adults with learning difficulties. In most cases only the keywords from the spoken message are signed rather than every word.

	British Sign Language	Signed English	Makaton Vocabulary	Signalong	Communica-tion Link
Home	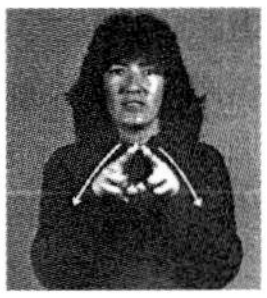	As BSL	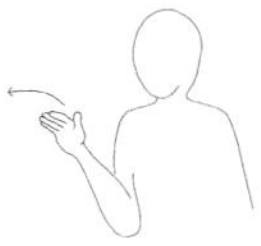	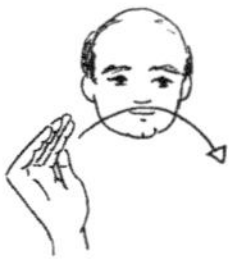	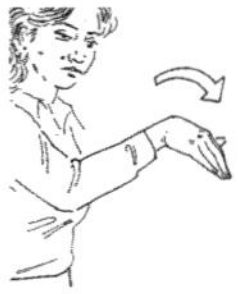
To go, advance	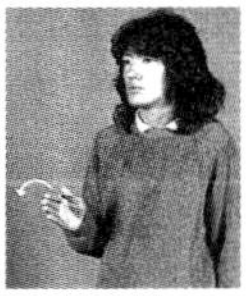	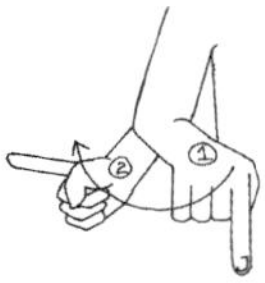	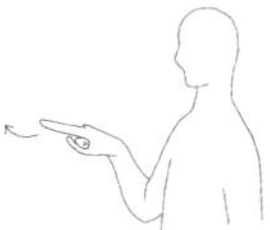	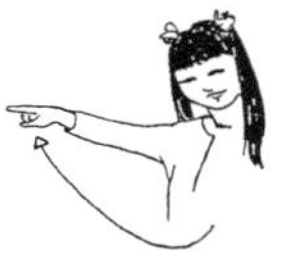	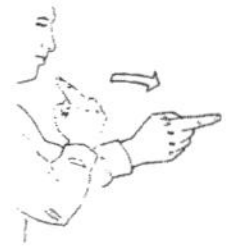
To want	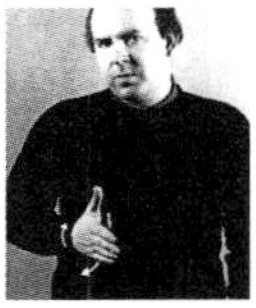	As BSL	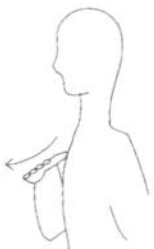	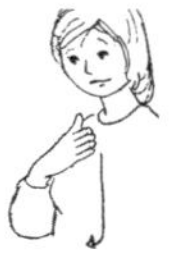	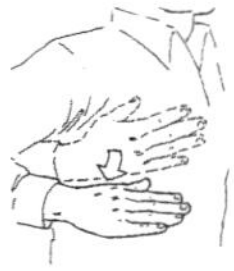
To tease	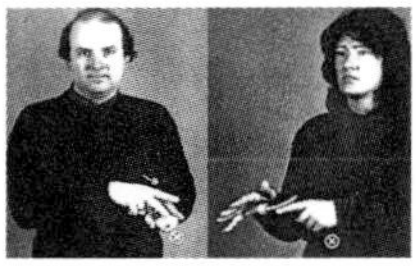	As BSL	As BSL	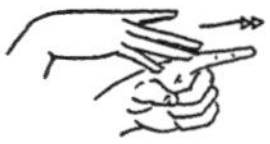	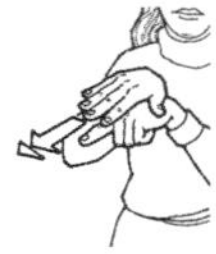
Tired	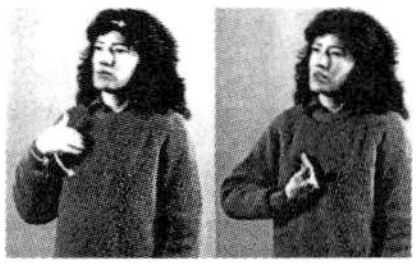	As BSL	As BSL	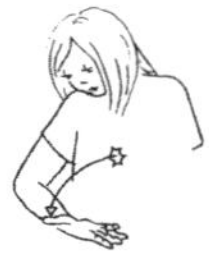	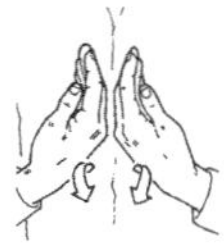
Noisy	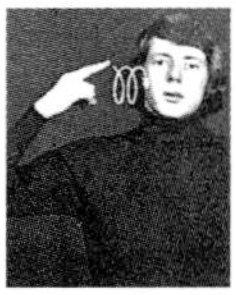	As BSL	As BSL	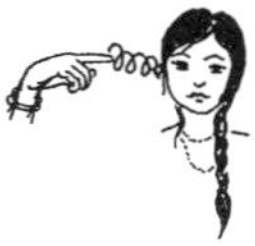	As BSL
Because	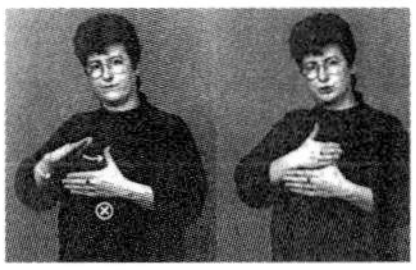	As BSL	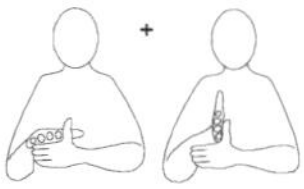	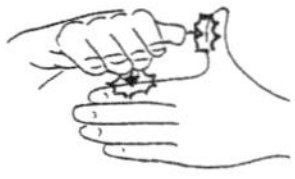	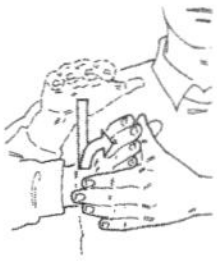
But	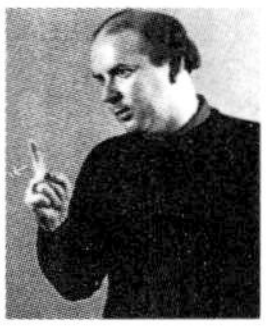	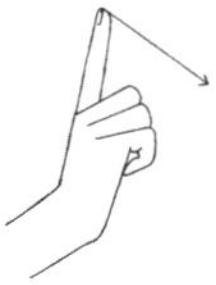	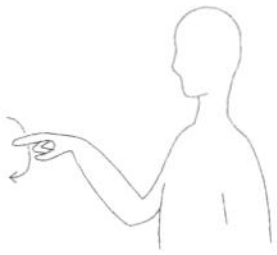	As BSL	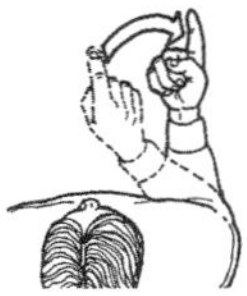

Fig. 10.1. Comparison of signs across the various signing systems.

Signalong, another sign vocabulary developed in the UK, has approximately 2000 signs which cover all aspects of vocabulary from that which is particularly relevant for young children to vocabulary related to the work place. As with the Makaton Vocabulary, new sets of vocabulary are produced as required. It is used primarily with children and adults with learning disabilities and has been used to extend the signed vocabulary of those using the Makaton Vocabulary.

Paget–Gorman Signed Speech is a sign system that aims to provide an accurate representation of spoken English and makes no claims to being a language in its own right with a separate grammar. The function of basic signs is to represent groups of words with a common concept. There are instructions for over 4000 signs, but with the use of affixes this can be greatly increased.

In countries other than the UK vocabularies or sign systems may have been developed from the relevant national sign language, *e.g.* Signed Norwegian from Norwegian Sign Language.

Comparisons of signs across the various signing systems are shown in Figure 10.1.

Graphic symbol systems and sets

There are a variety of graphic symbols available. These divide into two categories: pictographic sets that represent vocabulary in a concrete fashion, and symbol systems that are more abstract.

Picture or symbol sets are basically closed sets (or if they are expanded they are done so with no clearly defined rules beyond extending the vocabulary). Symbol systems have rules for expansion of vocabulary or of grammatical structures beyond the existing system. Symbol systems are characterized by having a logical internal structure, which is reasonably consistent across different categories of meaning and grammar.

Selection of one type of graphic system or set should not preclude use of symbols from another. A child may have a core vocabulary from one system/set, with symbols from another set imported as required, *e.g.* for specific topics or special interests. Difficulties can arise when children and adults transfer from one environment to another if the new environment does not support the user's existing AAC system. In instances such as this it is essential that the user should not be disadvantaged by having to learn a new language, which would be comparable to speaking adults having to learn a foreign language. Therefore, in new environments or when changes are made to an individual's communication system, professionals should *never* remove what the user already knows.

The range of symbols now available is considerably greater than even 10 years ago, and use of established symbol systems has changed. For example, the greater variety of symbols has meant that AAC users can have cognitively appropriate graphic representations of the words they need. As a result, the use of systems such as Blissymbols has declined as there has been a huge swing towards the use of visually representational symbols, *e.g.* Picture Communication Symbols (PCS). However, the meaning of these simpler symbols is context-dependent, so the meaning can change according to the context.

Professionals and researchers are now considering the lack of transparency in graphic symbol systems when devising the vocabulary required by their clients. This is ensuring that appropriate symbol sets and/or systems are selected to meet the AAC user's vocabulary needs.

Research has shown that output produced by AAC users who also have some intelligible speech, is different depending on the mode of expression, and Smith (1996) observed that "In most cases, PCS output was 'reduced', relative to spoken output, essentially consisting of single-PCS utterances, sometimes strung together . . ."

The graphic symbols in a communication book or on a chart represent the vocabulary available to the user. Symbols can be recognized rather than recalled, which may benefit those with learning difficulties. Children who sign may also need the support of symbols to communicate with people who do not understand signing. Graphic symbols can be of benefit to those developing literacy skills as they provide a bridge between symbols and text, or provide an alternative to text for children with specific difficulties in learning to read.

As with manual signing, symbols can provide support for listeners who are struggling to interpret speech of poor intelligibility.

Points to consider when selecting a graphic pictorial/symbolic communication system include:

- Is the graphic set/system easily understood? Does the user respond to concrete pictures?
- Does the graphic system contain all the necessary vocabulary? How flexible is the vocabulary and how can be it be expanded?
- What is the relationship of the graphic system to spoken English? Is it necessary to point to each item or can the length of the message be reduced by indicating key symbols or pictures?
- Does the system/set match the user's ability, age and language experience?
- Does the system contain sufficient strategies for expanding the vocabulary without greatly increasing the number of items to be accessed?
- Words should always be presented with symbols or pictures so the listener does not have to have any knowledge of the graphic symbols to understand the user's message.
- Large graphic symbol charts or books may not be very portable, but topically organized boards or communication books can be used in situations where a larger chart is impractical. Some users will need a core vocabulary, with additional topical vocabulary available in specific situations.
- As graphic systems can be accessed through eye-pointing they are ideally suited to those with severe physical limitations.
- Use of graphic symbols will inevitably reduce the rate of communication, therefore, the user's output is likely to be telegrammatic, *i.e.* abbreviated: "I see sister baby dog".
- The nature of graphic symbols systems, and the way in which they are processed, may also contribute to differences in output, when compared to speech (Smith 1996).
- The abstract nature of symbols will allow a user to convey a wider range of meanings than pictorial sets, but they may be more difficult to understand and learn in the initial stages.
- The graphic symbol set/system selected should ideally meet both immediate and long-term communication goals.

- Issues such as the expectations of communication partners, and the symbols already in use in an environment, need to be considered.

PICTURE SETS

There are closed sets of vocabulary that attempt to translate words into a highly representational graphic format. However, the assumption that all these symbols are transparent has proved erroneous. When faced with a sheet of graphic symbols without text, it can be as difficult as trying to guess the meaning in a complex Blissymbol if one knows no Bliss!

A number of picture sets have been created for use with children and adults who have communication difficulties. They aim to provide a direct representation of a finite vocabulary. Generally speaking, they are of more use to young and less cognitively able communicators. However, young children may well begin with pictures, and at a later stage have new vocabulary introduced from a symbol system.

Points to consider when selecting a picture set include:
- Some users may need coloured pictures, *e.g.* PCS or Pick'n'Stick, rather than black and white pictures. Others may find colour confusing.
- Some picture sets have larger vocabularies than others, *e.g.* PCS has 3000 symbols, Pick'n' Stick only about 800.
- Some sets use complex pictures, *i.e.* may be highly representational, but are hard to draw, *e.g.* PCS.
- Pictures may be more visually confusing for those with visual or visual perceptual difficulties.
- Care needs to be taken when creating charts or pages for a communication book, to avoid visual confusion.
- Some picture sets may be more acceptable for older users, *e.g.* Pick'n'Stick.

There is a limited number of picture sets available, the most popular being PCS because of the clarity of the symbols and the extensive vocabulary. It is used primarily with children, although it is suitable for adults with learning difficulties. Johnson (1981) states in her manual that PCS is most appropriate "for use with persons for whom a simple level of expressive language is acceptable. Typically this involves a limited vocabulary and moderately short sentence structures." The option to have either black and white or colour symbols is useful both in PCS and Pick'n'Stick.

Pictogram Symbols provide a completely different perspective as this system comprises white symbols on a black background. This is thought to help attract the user's attention to the symbol. It may also be useful for children and young people with visual difficulties, although some of the symbols appear to be quite abstract. These symbols are used widely in Scandinavia with a range of users.

Pick'n'Stick (colour) and Touch'n'Talk (black and white) are clear drawings that represent a wide variety of common vocabulary. Packs of words accompany the pictures, although any appropriate word could be used instead. These pictures are relatively transparent and could provide a useful basis for a communication system for those with more complex difficulties.

Symbol Systems

There are a number of different symbol systems that have varied in their development and use. Historically, each symbol system was seen as an important single entity that should not be 'corrupted' by the inclusion of symbols from another system. Therefore, specific graphic symbol systems tended to be chosen because they fitted in with environmental philosophy, *e.g.* only Makaton or only Rebus would be used. Teachers and therapists have often based their decisions on selection of graphic symbol systems for their clients on either the widely available training (*e.g.* Makaton Vocabulary), or software for writing (*e.g.* Writing with Symbols). However, this view is changing due to the availability of additional symbol systems in appropriate graphic formats for the computer. Many environments now recognize a 'needs led' rather than a 'system led' approach to ensure the needs of the individual are being met. This reflects a greater understanding of how AAC users learn and use their expressive means of communication.

Points to consider when selecting a symbol system include:

- Does the system offer the breadth of vocabulary required?
- How easy are the symbols to draw quickly if necessary?
- Will the AAC user need to use grammar in her/his utterances, *e.g.* will s/he need to represent every word and word ending via symbols? If so, are the graphic representations as meaningful and adequate as possible?
- Are there facilities for the user to generate new meanings from existing symbols?

Of the variety of symbol systems available, the most commonly used in the UK are Rebus and Makaton symbols. Although Rebus symbols have been in existence for many years (as the Peabody Rebus Reading Scheme), they share a common core vocabulary with Makaton symbols. However, the two systems have developed in different directions. For example, at present Rebus contains more vocabulary for adults with learning difficulties, whereas the Makaton contains more vocabulary for the more cognitively able child (with the National Curriculum Vocabulary), although it too is now developing more functional vocabulary for those with learning difficulties.

Picsyms and Compic are lesser-used symbol systems. Both allow for the creation of new symbols by following their respective guidelines. Compic symbols were specifically designed and created for the computer and the software was amongst the first AAC software available. Both these symbol systems are generally more abstract than Rebus and Makaton, and the use of dotted lines in Picsyms can make the symbols particularly difficult to interpret.

Sigsymbols were developed in an attempt to provide the classroom teacher with immediate access to new vocabulary without having to refer to a dictionary. Many of the symbols are line drawings and reasonably easy to interpret. Others are 'sign linked' symbols where the graphic representation is a line drawing of the manual sign. The manual signs are taken from British Sign Language (BSL) and used in a sign support English structure. Sigsymbols were designed to supplement signing as some children were unable to sign accurately due to physical difficulties.

Other symbol systems in use around the world include Oakland Schools Picture Dictionary, Talking Pictures, Self Talk, and DynaSyms (as used on the Dynavox voice output communication aid).

Blissymbolics was one of the first graphic symbol systems to be used with individuals who required augmentative communication. Although it was originally designed as an international language, it never received that status until used with non-speaking children with cerebral palsy. Since 1971, Blissymbols have been used worldwide for those who are cognitively able and require AAC. Blissymbols have some features of a *language* as they are composed of different elements in the same way as written words are composed of letters and spoken words are composed of sounds. New vocabulary can be generated easily through the use of 'special symbols' that mark novel words. For young cognitively able children, the addition of 'embellishments' to the basic symbol can make the symbol more representative of its meaning. This mechanism for increasing the transparency of the symbol is quite acceptable. Embellishments are added in a paler colour to avoid obscuring the basic symbol.

Comparisons of graphic symbols used across the various symbol systems are shown in Figure 10.2.

Tangible symbols
'Tangible symbols' or 'objects of reference' are not a formal communication system as such, but are used with an increasing number of children with severe learning disabilities as well as those with a dual sensory impairment. Rowland and Schweigert (1989) discuss the use of tangible symbols, which they subdivide into four categories: real objects, miniature objects, partial objects, and artificially associated textured symbols (this latter category will be discussed as tactile symbols). This type of approach has to be personalized as each individual may have a different referent for the same activity. For example, one AAC user may have a cup to represent a drink, another a toy cup, and a third may have the handle. Another example might be that one user has a piece of swimming hat to represent 'swimming', another may have a piece of swimsuit and another a piece of towel.

Tactile symbols are abstract tactile representations of words, or artificially associated and textured symbols (Rowland and Schweigert 1989). For example, a piece of cotton wool might represent 'activities', a paper clip could represent 'drinks', etc. They may be necessary in order to provide a client with limited vision access to a large vocabulary. However, this would be difficult to achieve in a communication book or chart as it is likely that there will be many tactile symbols required by the user. There would need to be a 'key' to the codes unless the tactile symbols were used on a voice output communication aid where the user would select symbols appropriate to the word or message to obtain a spoken message.

Readers wishing to obtain further information about sign and graphic symbol systems are advised to contact the local chapter of the International Society for Augmentative and Alternative Communication (Appendix 10.1) or the relevant national professional body for speech and language therapists (Appendix 10.2). For an overview of symbols systems, see Glennen and DeCoste (1997), Beukelman and Mirenda (1998) and Von Tetzchner and Martinsen (2000).

Speech output devices/voice output communication aids
Speech output devices or voice output communication aids (VOCAs) are a relatively new development in the field of AAC. They have been seen as the most important method of

	Pick'n'Stick	Pictogram Symbols	Picture Communication Symbols	Rebus
Home	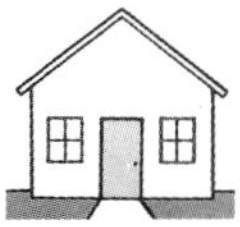	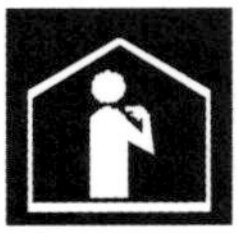	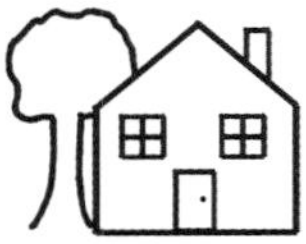	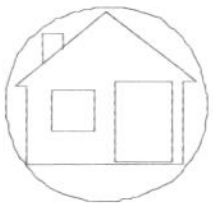
To go, advance	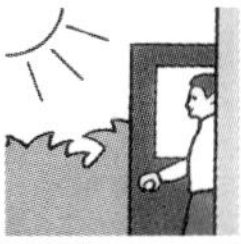	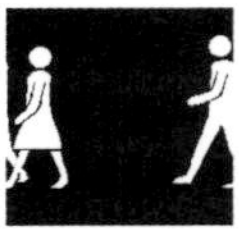	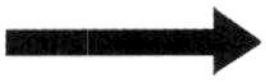	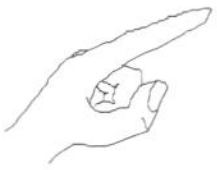
To want	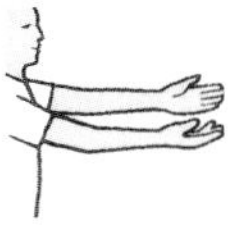		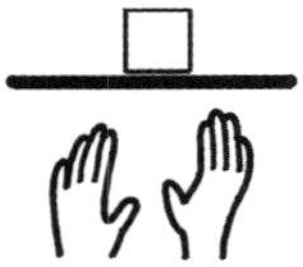	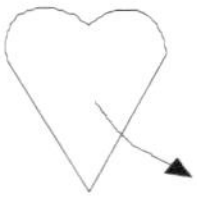
To tease	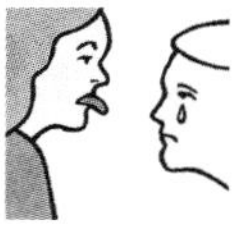	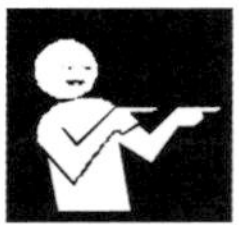		
Tired	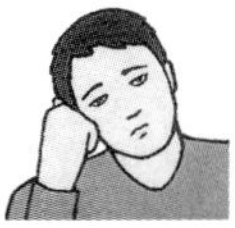	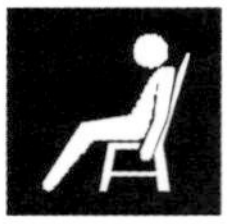	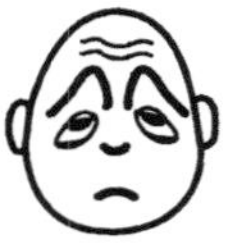	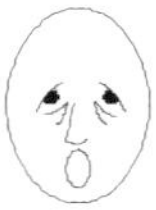
Noisy	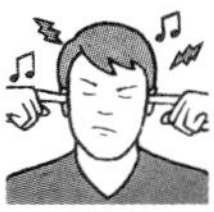			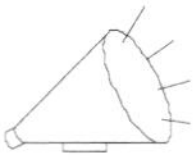
Because				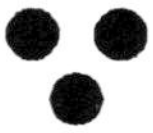
But				

Fig. 10.2. Comparison of graphic symbols

Makaton Vocabulary	Sigsymbols	Compic	Blissymbols	
	Draw as sign linked symbol	home		Home
		go (ambulant)		To go, advance
		want		To want
	Draw as sign linked symbol			To tease
	Draw as sign linked symbol	tired		Tired
	Draw as sign linked symbol			Noisy
	Draw as sign linked symbol			Because
	Draw as sign linked symbol			But

across the various symbol systems.

TABLE 10.1
Features of voice output communication aids (VOCAs)

Speech output	
Digitized output	Instantly recorded human speech
Synthesized output	Computer generated speech
Digitized/synthesized	
Displays	
Static displays	Fixed overlays (symbol or text) that do not change when a selection is made by the AAC user
Dynamic displays	The screen may change when a selection is made by the AAC user
Systems	
Dedicated systems	A device that is used as a stand-alone VOCA and cannot be used for other purposes (computer emulation may be possible with some dedicated devices)
Integrated systems	A device that can be used for a variety of purposes such as word processing, drawing or environmental control
PC-based systems	Software packages designed for face-to-face communication

augmenting speech, because they provide just that—*speech*. However, the effort required by many children with severe physical disabilities to operate these devices, in addition to the effort of learning to access the vocabulary stored in the device, should not be underestimated.

Alternative means of access, such as a switch or joystick, are available for most devices if users are unable to finger point. Some devices provide direct access via optical head-pointers or head-mouse type devices (this is a pointer control device controlled through head movements) in addition to switch and joystick access. Determining the most appropriate method of accessing a VOCA must be an interdisciplinary task. It is likely that a VOCA will be used in certain situations, for example when the user is sitting in a wheelchair with switches, joystick or optical head-pointer in position. When s/he is relaxing, it may well be impossible to access the VOCA effectively, hence the need for the back-up of a sign or graphic symbol system.

VOCAs have historically been seen as more desirable than the use of symbol charts or books, and in fact have been viewed as the ultimate goal because they provide speech. However, the status assigned to VOCAs is often unrealistic, as even the most effective VOCA user will not be able to use their device all the time. AAC users quickly decide when it is appropriate to use the device or when signs or symbols are more effective and appropriate. The physical demands of using a VOCA may be enormous and therefore extremely tiring. Despite these difficulties, a VOCA can provide an effective means of communication for many AAC users in many situations.

VOCAs can be subdivided into various groups, providing, for instance, digitized and/or synthesized speech, static or dynamic displays, and dedicated or integrated systems, as detailed in Table 10.1.

The selection of VOCAs is a complex process. It is impossible to make decisions without the AAC user trying the device at least in an assessment (preferably independent of the supplier). Ideally, more complex devices need to be tried over a longer period of time to ensure that both the user and the environment can use the device effectively. In many communication aid centres it has become clear that complex devices need to be trialled for two to three months prior to a decision regarding purchase.

Points to consider when choosing a VOCA include:

- What is the device to be used for?
- Who will take responsibility for coordinating use of the device?
- Who will take responsibility for programming the device?
- Is the user ambulant or a wheelchair user?
- Does the user have a variety of seats and positions in which they need to communicate via a VOCA?
- What is the user's level of language ability and cognitive level?
- Is auditory scanning necessary to support the user's visual skills?
- How is the user going to access the device (keyboard, optical headpointer, switches, joystick, etc.)?
- Which type of speech output (digitized or synthesized) will be most easily understood by the user?
- Are languages other than English spoken in the user's environment? If so, this may affect the choice of device as digitized speech may be required in order to record speech in the user's first language.
- Should graphic symbols or text be used on overlays? If graphic symbols are to be used, should these be the same as the user's existing graphic symbol system or should the graphic symbols available with devices be used (*e.g.* Minsymbols, Dynasyms)?
- Is the user at the level of single message hits or can s/he either combine icons (*e.g.* Minspeak) or need a hierarchical system (*e.g.* Dynavox, Talking Screen for Windows)?
- What level of training and support is available from the supplier/manufacturer?
- What level of training and support is necessary to ensure effective learning and use of the VOCA within the community (home or school)?

The range and sophistication of equipment is increasing rapidly, although costs appear to remain constant. As the range of available VOCAs is constantly changing, any list of aids would soon become redundant. Readers wishing to investigate the available options are advised to contact the appropriate chapter of the International Society of Augmentative and Alternative Communication (see Appendix 10.1), who will be able to direct them to local communication aid suppliers. As befits a field in which technology plays a central role, the most reliable source of up-to-date information is the internet.

Computer software

Mainstream technologies are becoming increasingly used in the field of augmentative communication. As a result, the number of programmes specifically designed for AAC use is growing. This software runs on the main computer platforms, Windows (including CE) and Macintosh. Some of the software contains the facility for writing as well as communication, and many programmes have vocabulary applications for different users. It is also possible to enable the user to launch other software from the communication software. For example, the user may want to draw or play a game instead of talking.

Some communication software packages also provide the facility to 'translate' from one symbol system to another. So if a chart has been created for a Blissymbol user and the same vocabulary is needed for a PCS user, then this can be quickly and easily accomplished. It is possible, in many of the programmes, to edit symbols either within the programme or via a separate drawing package.

Software is currently under development that will let the AAC user write and receive e-mail in symbols. This technology will open up new opportunities for AAC users.

Conclusion

This chapter has aimed at providing an overview of the factors to consider in selecting AAC systems for children with severe speech impairments. The use of AAC systems does not preclude existing methods of communication. Each mode of communication has its own value and will support unaided means of communication. The AAC user will learn when to use which method of communication, and will combine modes as necessary in order to communicate effectively.

In order to provide the AAC user with an effective means of communication, it is essential to introduce AAC at an early stage. Many children do not begin to use AAC until they start school at the age of 2 or 3 years or, in many instances, much later than this. Children are exposed to spoken language at an earlier age than this, so those who might need AAC should be introduced to signs and symbols as early as possible. Available research suggests this will not delay the development of speech in any way, although there are still many questions regarding the development of understanding and expression in non-speaking children.

"It will be clear that implementing a symbol programme for one user, or for a whole group of users . . . is a wide ranging and hugely time-consuming undertaking. . . Using symbols for communication and learning requires a commitment throughout the whole establishment" (Millar and Larcher 1998). The amount of work and effort required to ensure that an individual has an effective communication system should not be underestimated. However, following an interdisciplinary assessment to determine which AAC system will best meet the individual's needs, it is essential to ensure that "[the] vocabulary of each AAC system should be open-ended" (Glennen and deCoste 1997). Vocabulary must be motivating, stimulating and meet the needs of the user for any AAC system to be used effectively.

REFERENCES

Beukelman D., Mirenda P. (1992) *Augmentative and Alternative Communication: Management of Severe Communication Disorders in Children and Adults*. Baltimore: Paul Brooks.
—— —— (1998) *Augmentative and Alternative Communication: Management of Severe Communication Disorders in Children and Adults. 2nd Edn*. Baltimore: Paul Brookes.
Glennen S., DeCoste D. (1997) *Handbook of Augmentative and Alternative Communication*. San Diego: Singular Publishing.
Johnson, R. (1981) *The Picture Communication Symbols*. Solana Beach, CA: Mayer Johnson.
Millar S., Larcher J. (1998) *Symbol Software*. Edinburgh: CALL Centre.
Rowland, C., Schweigert, P. (1989) 'Tangible symbols: symbolic communication for individuals with multi-sensory impairments.' *Augmentative and Alternative Communication*, **5**, 226–34.

Smith, M. (1996) 'The medium or the message: A study of speaking children using communication boards.' *In:* Von Tetzchner, S., Jensen, M.H. (Eds) *Augmentative and Alternative Communication: European Perspectives*. London: Whurr, pp. 119–36.

Von Tetzchner, S., Martinsen, H. (2000) *Introduction to Augmentative and Alternative Communication. 2nd Edn*. London: Whurr.

APPENDIX 10.1

International Societies for Augmentative and Alternative Communication

ISAAC—CANADA
49 The Donway West, Suite 308
Toronto, ON, M3C 3M9
Canada
Tel: +1 416 385-0351
Fax: +1 416 385-0352
E-mail: secretariat@isaac-online.org
Website: http://www.isaac-online.org

ISAAC—DANMARK
Mogens Hygum Jensen
DPU
173, Skolebakken
Esbjerg OE, DK-6705
Denmark
Tel: +45 7514 1722
Fax: +45 7514 3168
E-mail: mogens@dpu.dk
Website: http://www.isaac.dk

ISAAC—GSC
Susanne Bünk
Pfarrer-Dr Hoffmann Str. 5a
53343 Wachtberg
Germany
Tel/Fax: +49 2225 9099317
E-mail: geschaeftsstelle@isaac-online.de
Website: http://www.isaac-online.de

ISAAC—IRELAND
c/o Paula Browne
Speech and Language Therapist
Cerebral Remedial Clinic
Vernon Avenue
Clantarf
Dublin 3
Ireland
Tel: +353 1 8057511
Fax: +353 1 8335496
E-mail: pbrowne@crc.ie

ISAAC—ISRAEL
c/o Judy Seligman-Wine
PO Box 40012
Mevasseret Zion 90805
Israel
Tel: +972 2 5335136
Fax: +972 2 5340581
E-mail: winej@netvision.net.il

ISAAC—NF (Netherlands/Flanders)
Secretariaat
Crailoseweg 116
1272 EX Huizen
The Netherlands
Website: http://www.isaac-nf.nl
E-mail: isaac-nf@wirehub.nl

ISAAC—NORWAY
Aina Ask
Hjelpemiddelsentralen i Hordaland
PB 121 Kokstad
5863 Bergen
Norway
Tel/Fax: +47 55 52 68 56
E-mail: aiask@hms.hl.no
Website: http://www.isaac.no/

ISAAC—SPAIN
C/Velez de Guevara 38 Bajo
(Plaza Escocia)
26005-Logrono-La Rioja
Spain
Tel: +34 941 581 582
Fax: +34 941 584 022
E-mail: administracion@isaac-es.org
Website: www.isaac-es.org

ISAAC—SUOMI-FINLAND ry.
Toimisto
Hämeenkatu 5 A
33100 Tampere
Finland
Tel: +358 3 260 3600
Fax: +358 3 260 3700
E-mail: isaacsuomifin@yritys.tpo.fi
Website: http://yritys.soon.fi/isaacsuomifin/
    index.htm

ISAAC—SVERIGE
c/o Kerstin Lorstrom
Salgvagen 24
Mora S-792-52
Sweden
Tel: +46 250 263 50
Fax: +46 250 380 44
E-mail: kerstin.mora@mail10.calypso.net

ISAAC—UK (Communication Matters)
c/o The ACE Centre
92 Windmill Road
Headington
Oxford OX3 7DR
England
Tel: +44 (0)870 606 5463
Fax: +44 (0)131 555 3279
E-mail: admin@communicationmatters.org.uk
Website: http://www.communicationmatters.
  org.uk

USSAAC
c/o Beatrice Bruno
Acting Managing Director
PO Box 21418
Sarasota
FL 34276
USA
Tel/Fax: +1 941 312 0992
E-mail: USSAAC@aol.com
Website: http://www.ussaac.org

APPENDIX 10.2

Professional bodies with responsibility for speech and language therapists

Australia
Speech Pathology Australia
2nd Floor, 11–19 Bank Place
Melbourne
VIC 3000
Australia
Tel: +61 3 9642 4899
Fax: +61 3 9642 4922
E-mail: office@speechpathologyaustralia.org.au
Website: http://www.speechpathologyaustralia.
  org.au

Canada
Canadian Association of Speech–Language
  Pathologists
200 Elgin Street, Suite 401
Ottawa
Ontario K2P 1L5
Tel: +1 613 567 9968 *or* +1 800 259 8519
Fax: +1 613 567 2859
E-mail: caslpa@caslpa.ca
Website: www.caslpa.ca

New Zealand
New Zealand Speech–Language Therapists
  Association (NZSTA)
Suite 369, 63 Remuera Road
Newmarket
Auckland
New Zealand
Tel: +64 3 235 8257
Fax: +64 3 235 8850
E-mail: nzsta@clear.net.nz
Website: http://www.nzsta-speech.org.nz

South Africa
South African Speech–Language–Hearing
  Association
PO Box 91042
Auckland Park 2006
South Africa
Tel: +27 11 726 5014
Fax: +27 11 726 5013
E-mail: saslha@mweb.co.za
Website: http://www.saslha.org.za

UK
Royal College of Speech and Language Therapists
2/3 White Hart Yard
London SE1 1NX
Tel: +44 (0)20 7378 1200
Fax: +44 (0)20 7403 7254
E-mail: postmaster@rcslt.org
Website: http://www.rcslt.org

USA
American Speech–Language–Hearing
  Association (ASHA)
10801 Rockville Pike
Rockville
MD 20852
Tel: +1 800 321 ASHA or +1 498 2071
Fax: +1 877 541 5035
E-mail: actioncenter@asha.org
Website: http://professional.asha.org

INDEX

(Page numbers in *italics* refer to figures/tables.)

A

Access, 140
Action Plan, 117, *118*
Active vocabulary, 2
ADHD, *see* Attention deficit hyperactivity disorder
Adolescence
    issues in, 124–135
    case studies
        body image, 132
        competence, effect of self-esteem on, 129–131
        conflict and move towards independence, 131
        disability, coming to terms with, 127–129
        multiple reasons for restricted use, 134–135
        parental separation, 127
        protective factors for mental health/parental influence, 125–127
    learning difficulties, 132–134
    private vocabulary, 127
Aided communication, 96–98, 162
Aided Language Stimulation (ALS), 120–121
Airflow in speech production, 42
Airway, occlusion, *45*
Alexander's disease, and pseudobulbar palsy, 59
American Sign Language (ASL), 163
Anatomy of emotion, 28–29
Angelman syndrome, 23
Aphasia, 67
    Broca's, 35
        speech, 38–39
    central, 25
    fluent, 2
    receptive, 23–25, 67
    Wernicke's, 25
Articulation, 44
Articulatory dyspraxia, 49–50
Asperger syndrome, 25, 67
Assessment, 62, 73–86
    activities, 76
    cognitive, 77–78
    of communication environment, 83–85
    of general health, 81
    of hearing, 77
    of language comprehension, 78–79
    of literacy, 79–80
    methods, 75–76
    of motor skills, 76
    paediatric, 68
    setting, 74–75

    of speech, 80–81
    of vision, 77
Ataxia
    slowed speech development, 48
Ataxia–telangiectasia, dysarthria, 61
Athetosis, dysarthria in, 58
    Auburtin, early experiments of, 15
Attention deficit hyperactivity disorder (ADHD), 68
Audiometry, 62
Auditory agnosia, 10
    in Landau–Kleffner syndrome, 27
Auditory association area, *see under* Brain
Auditory scanning, 154–156
Augmentative and alternative communication (AAC)
    access, 140
    Action Plan, 117, *118*
    assessment for, *see* Assessment
    auditory scanning, partner assisted, 154–156
    in Australia, 138
    in autism, 83
        case history, 156–158
    Blissymbols, 153, 158, 165, 167, 169, *171*
    camps, 147
    charitable funding, 143
    choice, for schools, 114–115
    communication partners, 84, 121
        training/support, 144
    computerized, 69
        funding, 115
        see also Computers
    coordinator, 112
    creating materials, 118
    development of new technology, 142–143
    funding for, 85, 110, 143
        charitable, 143
    graphic symbols, *see* Symbol systems
    head mouse, 130, 172
    head switches, 155, 159–160, 172
    input system, 69
    integration with other systems, 139–141
    International Society of Augmentative and Alternative Communication (ISAAC), 145, 176–177
    internet resources, 145, 173
        AAC organizations, 176–177
        listservs, 145
    introduction into home, 92–94
    listservs, 145
    and literacy, 121
    manual systems, 162–165

models of service delivery, 137–139
mounting, 140
objects of reference, 169
organization of services, 137–139
organizations, 145, 176–177
output system, 69
paediatric assessment, 69–70
picture systems, *see* Picture systems
policies towards, 84
possible roles, 69
primary service, 138–139, 145
in rural areas, 138, 139, 145–147
secondary service, 139, 145–146
selecting a system, basic considerations, 162
semantic compaction, 126
service delivery, three-tier model, 138–139, 145–
    147
sign languages, *see* Sign languages
specialists, 112–113
support organizations, 145, 176–177
symbol systems, *see* Symbol systems
tactile symbols, 169
tangible symbols, 169
team, 73–74, 111–114, 137
technological support, 84
tertiary service, 139, 146–147
training for school staff, 110–111
transport, 141
visual impairment, 154–156
voice output communication aids, *see* Voice out-
    put communication aids
wheelchair users, 139, 172
    case histories, 125–127, 129–131, 132, 134–
        135, 158–161
Augmented Communication Online Users Group
    (ACOLUG), 145
Australian Group on Severe Communication Impair-
    ment (AGOSCI), 145
Autism/autistic spectrum disorder
    AAC and, 67, 83
        case history, 156–158
    assessment, 78
    echolalia, 2
    and hearing, 77
    in Landau–Kleffner syndrome, 27
    learning disability, 30
    pathological basis, 12
    receptive dysprosodia, 29, 30
    specific language impairment, 25
    use of communication book, 98
    use of objects to aid communication, 97
    use of signing, 95

B

Basal ganglia, *see under* Brain
Batten's disease, and pseudobulbar palsy, 59

Bilateral perisylvian syndrome, 59
Blissymbols, 153, 158, 165, 167, 169, *171*
    use in cerebral palsy, 169
Body image in adolescence, 131–132
Braille, 22
Brain
    association areas, 17–19
        auditory, 10–12
        visual, 18
    basal ganglia function, 41–42
    Broca's motor speech area, 12–14, *15*, 33–36
        in articulatory dyspraxia, 49
        lateralization, 35–36
    bulbar function, 52–54
        dysfunction, *55*
    cerebellar function, 39–42
    cerebral dominance, 19–20
    cortex, Brodman's map, 16, *17*
    extrapyramidal system, 28, 29
    injury, traumatic, 68
    planum temporale, 10–14
    hemispheres, functions of right/left, *18*
    Heschl's gyrus, 7, *8*, *11*, 16, *35*
    imaging, 62
    limbic system, 28
    nuclei of pons and medulla, *53*
    Temporal lobe, *11*
    Wernicke's area, 10, 12, *14*, *15*, 18, 33
British Sign Language (BSL), 163, *164*
Broca's aphasia, 35, 38–39
Broca's motor speech area, *see under* Brain
Brodman's map of the cortex, 16, *17*
Bulbar function, *see under* Brain
Bulbar palsy, 56–58
    ataxic, 61
    causes, *56*
    dyskinetic, 59–61
        hyperkinetic, 60–61
        hypokinetic, 59
    in Prader–Willi syndrome, 58
    Worster Drought type, *38*
    see also Pseudobulbar palsy

C

Cameleon, 125, 154, 159, 160
Case studies, 125–127, 128–132, 134–135, 153–161
Central deafness, 10
Central hearing, 6–10
Cerebellar function, 39–42
Cerebellar mutism, 41
Cerebral palsy
    with dysarthria, 58
    with dysphonia, 43
    hyperkinetic, 30
    need for AAC, 65–66
    with pseudobulbar palsy, 59

use of AAC
case studies, 125–135, 153–156
model, 145–147
use of Blissymbols, 169
with visual impairment, 154–156
Child abuse, 3
Chromosomal analysis, 62
Cleft palate syndrome, *51*
AAC, 68
dysarthria, 51
Cluttering, 42
'Cocktail party' speech, 12
Cocktail party syndrome, 2
Cognition, 20–21
assessment, 77–78
Communication
aided, 96–98
technology, funding, 115
environment, assessment of, 83
in school
creating opportunities, 119–120
intervention approach, 98–100
nonverbal, 27–30, 133
opportunities, 83
Communication book/diary, 97–98
Communication Link, *164*
Communication Matters (ISAAC-UK), 145, 177
Communication partners, training, 84, 144
in schools, 121
Communication support teacher, 112
Communicative competence, development of, *82*
Communicative interaction in home, 93
Compic, 168, *171*
Computers, 69, 139, 168
Cameleon, 125, 130–131, 154, 159, 160
funding, 115
laptop, 141
software, 173–174
EZ Keys, 126, 130, 154
Switch Clicker, 155–156
Talking Screen, 125–126
Writing With Symbols, 168
touch screen, 125
Cortical evoked responses, 62
Curriculum, national, 116

D

Darwin, Charles, 28
Deaf–blind children, 22
Deaf children, 22
Deafness
central, 10
conductive, 5
sensorineural, *4*, 5–6
and learning disability, 67
Degenerative disorders, 68–69

Delayed speech development, 47–50
male predominance, 48
Deprivation, psychosocial, 3
Developmental disability team, 137
Developmental speech and language disorders, 67–68
Developmental speech retardation syndrome, 23–25
Disability
coming to terms with, 127–128
case study, 128–129
social model, 148–150
DNA testing, 62
Down syndrome
developmental speech disorder, 48
dysphonia, 43
learning disability, 66
use of signing, 94
Drooling, in ataxic bulbar palsy, *61*
Dysarthria, 50–52, 68
anatomical causes, 51
extrapyramidal, 59–60
forms of, *50*
neurological, 51–52
spastic, 58
Dyskinesia, 60
Dyslexia, pathological basis, 12
Dysphasia
acquired receptive, 25
developmental semantic, 23–25
epileptic, 25–27
expressive, 37
acquired, 37–39
in Landau–Kleffner syndrome, 27
receptive
acquired, 25
in Landau–Kleffner syndrome, 27
Dysphonia, 43
neurological, 44
Dysplasia, opercular, 59
Dyspraxia, 68
AAC, 68
articulatory, 49–50
Dysprosodia, 10
expressive, 29
receptive, 29, 30
Dystrophy, myotonic, 57–58

E

Ear, 5
Echolalia, 2, 12
Education
funding implications of AAC provision, 110
individualized education plan (IEP), 109, 116–117
special needs, 103–108
tertiary institutes, 144–145
see also School

Electrocochleography, 62
Encephalitis, and pseudobulbar palsy, 59
Environment
    communication, 83–85
    family, 90
    language, 3
    stimulation, 2–4
Environmental control units, 139
Epilepsy
    AAC, 68
    assessment of health, 81
    lateralization of speech processing, 36
    see also Landau–Kleffner syndrome
Epileptic dysphasia, 25–27
Expressive dysphasia, *see under* Dysphasia
Expressive dysprosodia, *see under* Dysprosodia

F
Facial palsy, *57*
Fahr syndrome, 61
Family
    breakdown, 127
    as communicative environment, 90
    as consumers, 90
    in crisis, 91
    as decision makers, 88
    as a system, 88
    as trainers, 91
Feeding difficulties
    assessment, 69
    in cerebral palsy, 66
Finger spelling, 163
Fragile X syndrome
    DNA testing for, 62
    echolalia, 2
    language involvement, 23
Friedreich's ataxia, and dysarthria, 61
Funding, 85, 110, 143
    charitable, 143

G
Gangliosidosis, and pseudobulbar palsy, 59
Glutaric aciduria, 61
Goldenhar syndrome, 43
Graphic symbols, *see* Symbol systems

H
Haemophilus influenzae, 6
Hallervorden–Spatz disease, 61
Hare lip, *51*
Hawking, Stephen, 134
Head injury, and pseudobulbar palsy, 59
Hearing
    assessment, 4, 69, 77
    central, 6–10
    peripheral, 4–6

Hearing impairment, 67
    see also Deafness
Hemiplegia, delayed speech maturation, 48
Herpes simplex encephalitis, and pseudobulbar palsy, 59
Heschl's gyrus, *see under* Brain
High frequency hearing loss, 5
Homunculus, 39, *40*
Huntingdon's chorea, 30
Hydrocephalus, cocktail party speech, 2
Hypercalcaemia, cocktail party speech, 2
Hypoglossal paralysis, *57*
Hypoxia–ischaemia, and pseudobulbar palsy, 59

I
Inclusion, 106
Independence, move towards, 131
Individualized education plan (IEP), 109, 116–117
Inner language, 1–2, 20–21, 133
Insertions, 47, 48
Intelligence, 22–23
International Society of Augmentative and Alternative Communication (ISAAC), 145, 173, 176–177
Internet resources, 145, 173
IQ, definition, 22

J
Jaw jerk reflex, 58

K
Kernicterus, 60
Kinaesthetic memory, 39, 44–46
Klinefelter syndrome, 23

L
Landau–Kleffner syndrome, 10, 25–27, 68
Language, 21
    comprehension assessment, 78
    environment, 3
    learning, environmental stimulation, 2
    see also Sign language
Larynx, 42–44
Learning, 14–20
    language, environmental stimulation, 2
    localization in the brain, 19
Learning disability, 66
    in autism, 30
    in Down syndrome, 66
Leigh's encephalopathy, 61
Lexicon, 10–14
    visual, 18
Lip-reading, 18
Literacy
    and AAC, 121
    assessment, 79–80
Lord Rayleigh's organ, 44, *45*

M

Maindumping, 106
Mainstream schools, 106–107
Makaton Vocabulary, 163, *164*, 168, *171*
Manual signing, 94–96, 162–165
    see also Sign language
Memory
    kinaesthetic, 39, 44–46
    short-term, 20–21
    see also Learning
Meningitis, bacterial, 6
Metachromatic leukodystrophy, and pseudobulbar
    palsy, 59
Middle ear disease, 5
Miller's organ pipes, *9*
Mitochondrial encephalopathy, 61
Moebius syndrome, 67
Motor engram, 44–46
Multiple disability, 154–156
Multiple sclerosis, and pseudobulbar palsy, 59
Muscle stretch reflexes, 58–61
Mutism
    in Broca's aphasia, 38
    cerebellar, 41
    in dysphasia, 25
    in Landau–Kleffner syndrome, 27
Myasthenia gravis, 44
Myotonic dystrophy, 57–58

N

National curriculum, 116
Neologisms, 25
    in Broca's aphasia, 39
Nonverbal communication, 27–30

O

Objects of reference, 169
Omissions, 47, 48
Opercular dysplasia, 59
Organ, of Lord Rayleigh, 44, *45*
Organ pipes, of D.C. Miller, *9*
Organization of AAC services, 137–139
Orofacial dyskinesia, 60
Oromotor difficulties, in cerebral palsy, 66
Otitis media, 5

P

Paget–Gorman Signed Speech, 165
Palatal function, 44
Paralysis, hypoglossal, *57*
Parental influence, 125–127
Parental separation, 127
Parkinsonism, 30, 42
    hypokinetic bulbar palsy, 59
Passive vocabulary, 1, 2
Peripheral hearing, 4–6

Phonagnosia, 10
Phonological development, 39–42
Pick'n'Stick, 167, *170*
Pictogram Symbols, 167, *170*
Picture cards, 153
Picture Communication Symbols (PCS), 157, 165–
    167, *170*
Picture Exchange Communication System (PECS),
    157
Picture systems, 69, 153, 165–167, *170–171*
    black and white *vs* colour, 167
    Pick'n'Stick, 167, *170*
    Pictogram Symbols, 167, *170*
    Picture Communication Symbols (PCS), 157,
        165–167, *170*
    Touch'n'Talk, 167
Planum temporale, *see under* Brain
Prader–Willi syndrome, 58
Primary language disorder, 2
Primitive feeding reflexes, 56
Profiling child's abilities, 81–83
Protective reflexes, 54
Pseudobulbar palsy, 58–59
Psychosocial deprivation, 3

R

Rayleigh, Lord, 44, *45*
Rebus symbols, 157, 168, *170*
Receptive aphasia, 23–25, 67
    see also Dysphasia, receptive
Receptive dysprosodia, 29
Reflexes
    muscle stretch, 58–61
    primitive feeding, *56*
    protective, 54
Repetitive strain injury (RSI), 76–77, 132
Reversals, 47, 48
Rhinophony, 42
Rural services, 138
    support to families, 144, 145–147

S

Saliva control, 69
    see also Drooling
School
    choice of AAC systems, 114–115
    communication support needs, 104–105
    inclusion, 106–107
    individualized education plan (IEP), 109, 116–117
    mainstream, 106–107
    models of provision, 107–108
    placements, 106–107
    special educational needs, 103–108
    special needs assistant (SNA), 113–114
    staff development, 114
    supportive environment, 108–115

training in AAC, 110–111
School Development Plan (UK), 110
Secondary speech disorder, 2
Segawa disease, bulbar palsy, 59
Self-esteem, effect of competence on, 129
   case study, 129–131
Semantic compaction, 126
Semantic–pragmatic disorder, 23–25
Semon's law, 42
Sensorineural deafness, 5–6
   audiogram, *4*
Service delivery, three-tier model, 138–139, 145–147
Severe Communication Impairment Outreach Project (SCIOP), 146
Short-term memory, 20–21
Signalong, 163, *164*, 165
Signing, manual, 94–96, 162–165
Sign languages, 94–95, 162, 163–165
   American, 163
   British, 163, *164*
   Communication Link, *164*
   comparisons, *164*
   deaf, 94–95
   finger spelling, 163
   Makaton Vocabulary, 163, *164*
   Norwegian, 165
   Paget–Gorman Signed Speech, 165
   Signalong, 163, *164*
   Signed English, *164*
Sign supported English, 163
Sigsymbols, 168, *171*
Social model of disability, 148–150
Software, *see under* Computers
Spastic dysarthria, 58
Special educational needs, 103–108
Special needs assistant (SNA), 113–114
Specific language impairment, 23–25
   differentiation from autism, 25
Speech
   assessment of, 80–81
   comprehensibility, 80
   cluttering, 42
   development
      delayed, 47–50
         in Down syndrome, 48
         male predominance, 48
      normal, 46–47
   insertions, 47
   and language disorders, developmental, 67–68
   motor learning, 39–42
   omissions, 47
   pathologists, 144, 147
   production, 42–62
      airflow, 42
      articulation, 44, *45*

      palatal function, 44
      voice, 42
   reversals, 47
   stuttering, 42
   substitutions, 47, 48
Speech and language development
   effect of child abuse on, 3
Speech and language therapists, 113
   professional bodies, 177
Spina bifida, 66
Stammering, 41, 67–68
Subacute sclerosing encephalitis, and pseudobulbar palsy, 59
Substitutions, 47, 48
Support organizations, 145, 176–177
Support services, 143–147
Support team *vs* support network, 111
Sydenham's chorea, 30
Symbolic function, 21–22
Symbol systems, 168–169
   Blissymbols, 153, 158, 165, 167, 169, *171*
   Compic, 168, *171*
   Makaton Vocabulary, 163, *164*, 168, *171*
   Picsyms, 168
   Picture Communication Symbols (PCS), 157, 165–167, *170*
   Picture Exchange Communication System (PECS), 157
   Rebus, 157, 168, *170*
   Sigsymbols, 168, *171*
Syntactical development, 33–39
   normal, 36–37
System for Augmenting Language (SAL), 120–121

T
Tactile symbols, 169
Tangible symbols, 169
Tardive dyskinesia, 60
TEACCH approach, 78
   in autism, 67
Team, 73–74, 137
   collaborative working, 84, 111–114
   developmental disability, 137
Technological support, 84
Telegrammatic speech
   in Broca's aphasia, 39
Tongue, hemiatrophy, *57*
Touch'n'Talk, 167
Tourette syndrome, 29
Training in AAC
   for communication partners, 84, 121, 144
   for family/community, 143–145
   for school staff, 110–111, 121
      accredited, 111
   for speech pathologists, 144
Transcortical aphasia, 14

Transport, 141
Treacher–Collins syndrome, 43, 67

U
Unaided communication, 162
United States Society for Augmentative and Alternative Communication (USSAAC), 145, 177

V
Velocardiofacial syndrome, 67
Verbal agnosia, 10
Verbal reasoning, 21
Video addict syndrome, 24
Video consultancy, 146
Videofluoroscopy, 53, 62
Video taping
 for AAC assessment, 75
 to guide intervention, 93–94
Videotelephony, 138
Vision, assessment of, 77
Visual impairment, 154–156
Vocabulary
 basic, 3
 core, 119
 fringe, 119
 pre-programmed, 119
 private, 127
 sets, 163–165
  Makaton, 163
Vocal cords, 42
Voice, 42–44

Voice output communication aids (VOCAs), 76, 98, 169–173
 accents
  lack of different, 142
  robotic, 153, 154
 access methods, 172
 BIGmack, 155
 DeltaTalker, 127
 DynaVox 2, 156
 Liberator, 126
 Lightwriter, 128–129, 154
 Minspeak, 126, 127
 RealVoice, 153, 158–159
 ScanPac, 159
 speed of communication, 134
 see also Computers

W
Wernicke–Geschwind model of speech, 14
Wernicke's dysphasia, 25
Wernicke's area, *see under* Brain
Wheelchair, 139, 140, 172
 AAC mounting, 140
 transport, 141
 users, case histories, 125–127, 129–131, 132, 134–135, 158–161
Williams syndrome, cocktail party speech, 2
Word board, 125
Word deafness, 10
 pathological basis, 12
Worster Drought palsy, *38*, 59, 67